Smoking Out the Barons:
The Campaign Against
the Tobacco Industry

Smoking Out the Barons:
The Campaign Against the Tobacco Industry

A Report of the British Medical Association
Public Affairs Division

A Wiley Medical Publication
Published on behalf of
The British Medical Association

JOHN WILEY & SONS
Chichester · New York · Brisbane · Toronto · Singapore

Library of Congress Cataloging in Publication Data:

Smoking out the barons: The Campaign against the tobacco industry

  (A Wiley medical publication)
  Includes index.
  1. Advertising—Cigarettes—Addresses, essays,
lectures. 2. Advertising—Cigarettes—Great Britain—
Addresses, essays, lectures. 3. Tobacco industry—
Great Britain—Addresses, essays, lectures.
I. British Medical Association. Public Affairs Division.
II. Series. [DNLM: 1. Advertising. 2. Health
Education—Great Britain. 3. Smoking—prevention &
control—Great Britain. QV 137 S6645]
HF6161.C35S66 1986   659.1'967973'0941   85-2614

ISBN 0 471 90937 8 (paper)

British Library Cataloguing in Publication Data:

British Medical Association. *Public Affairs Division*
  Smoking out the barons: The campaign against the tobacco industry.
  1. Tobacco—Physiological effect
  I. Title
  613.8'5   RA1242.T6

ISBN 0 471 90937 8

Printed and bound in Great Britain.

CONTENTS

LIST OF CONTRIBUTORS

Amanda Amos   *Senior Scientific Officer, Departments of
                          Health Education and Community Medicine,
                          Hampstead Health Authority, London, UK*

Simon Chapman   *Neil Hamilton Fairley Medical Research
                          Fellow, National Health and Medical
                          Research Council, Australia*

Nigel Duncan   *Deputy Editor of* Pulse, *London, UK*

Bobbie Jacobson   *Research Fellow in Health Promotion
                          London School of Hygiene and Tropical
                          Medicine, London, UK*

David Gilbert   *Social Audit, London, UK*

Frank Ledwith   *Department of Education, University
                          of Manchester*

Chapter 1

THE BMA'S CAMPAIGN AGAINST THE TOBACCO INDUSTRY

Nigel Duncan, Deputy Editor of *Pulse*

A CAMPAIGN IS HATCHED

On 16 October 1984 at a press conference in London, the British Medical Association launched the biggest campaign in its history to ban all tobacco advertising, sponsorship and promotion. It was to be the most prolonged and aggressive campaign ever undertaken by the Association and in identifying the tobacco industry as its principal target, the medical establishment was deliberately taking on what was probably the most insidiously powerful lobby in the country.

The BMA, a voluntary body representing 72 per cent of all practising doctors in the United Kingdom, had been closely involved in social reform ever since it was founded in 1832 and had played a large part in helping to bring about legislation on drink driving, the wearing of crash helmets and the compulsory wearing of seat belts. It had launched a campaign to ban boxing. However, surprisingly, it had never before set out to campaign against what was the single most avoidable cause of premature death and disease in the country—smoking.

Until 1984 the BMA had tended to do no more than try and persuade individual smokers to give up the habit. Now it was to launch a direct political assault on the giant multinational tobacco companies and their promotional activities which were being aimed directly at young people. Since research from the Office of Population Censuses and Surveys in 1983 had shown that £60 million worth of cigarettes were being sold to children under 16, it had to be assumed that the industry's promotional activities were succeeding.[1] Of the £150 million or so it was spending on promotion, some £15 million a

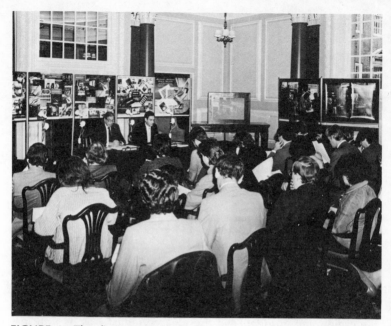

FIGURE 1   The first press conference in the campaign against the
tobacco industry, 16 October 1984.

year was going into sports sponsorship. The industry had diverted
much of its attention and resources in this direction, having been
forbidden by law since 1965 to advertise on television. Although the
number of cigarette brands involved in sports sponsorship in 1984 was
only 22, representing a mere 1.5 per cent of all companies sponsoring
sport, their television coverage amounted to about 30 per cent of the
total.[2] As with advertising and promotion, sports sponsorship was
governed by a voluntary agreement between the Tobacco Advisory
Council and the Government. However, it was clear that these agreements, due to expire at the end of 1985 and early in 1986, were not
working.

It was against this background that the BMA's campaign was born,
bringing the country's doctors directly into a fight which veteran anti-
smoking campaigners had been engaged in for 20 years, but even they
recognized that no-one knew more about the evidence of the dangers
of smoking than doctors.

But why had it taken the BMA so long to enter the arena? After all, the Royal College of Physicians had published four carefully documented reports highlighting the dangers of smoking, the first in 1962 and the most recent in November 1983. The BMA, too, had been passing resolutions at its annual representative meetings ever since 1965. What followed these resolutions had been more rhetoric than action, and what attempts the BMA had made to get more involved in the subject of smoking had been singularly unfruitful.

One of the most interesting of these attempts was in 1980 when representatives of the Association twice visited the Southampton research laboratories of British–American Tobacco Industries, the world's largest tobacco multinational. The first visit was as a result of a personal invitation to BMA secretary Dr John Havard from the company's managing director, whom he had met on holiday. Dr Havard accepted the invitation. He explained, 'I did so because I felt that if we went into a big anti-smoking campaign, it couldn't be said that the BMA didn't even accept an invitation to see what was going on'. He took with him Dr Frank Wells, a BMA under-secretary then respons- ible for the Association's Board of Science and Education, the commit- tee which deals with the scientific activities of the Association. The two men were entertained to lunch and were shown round the company's laboratories, which were engaged in research on trying to produce a less toxic cigarette. As a result of this, members of the Board of Sci- ence, under the chairmanship of Sir John Stallworthy, emeritus pro- fessor of obstetrics and gynaecology at Oxford University, were then invited to visit Southampton to discuss the issue of smoking at a meet- ing in the company's board room. Although there were those who questioned the wisdom of the BMA becoming so involved with a tobacco company, nothing that happened during these two visits per- suaded officials of the Association or members of the Board of Science to change their mind on BMA policy on smoking. 'We felt we were better informed', said Dr Wells, 'and if anything it hardened our line'. However, the visits were regarded as so sensitive that all references to them in the Association's draft annual report for that year were struck out by Dr Havard.

The next occasion on which the Board of Science attempted to tackle the issue of smoking was in 1982 when it considered a proposal to produce an anti-smoking leaflet *Help Others to Help Themselves Stop Smoking*. This was to be issued for use by anti-smoking self-help groups at work. The idea was principally the work of Dr John Dawson, who had by then taken over from Dr Wells as head of the BMA's Professional and Scientific division. He believed that if the leaflets persuaded just a few hundred people to give up smoking they would be worthwhile, but the response from the council of the BMA, the Association's ruling body, was distinctly lukewarm. Several members criticized the idea as ill-conceived. Dr Joe Kearns, chairman of the BMA's Occupational Health committee, warned that any suggestion that these anti-smoking groups should meet in working hours would upset employers.

When the campaigning organization ASH (Action on Smoking and Health) heard of the idea it was horrified. Its director, David Simpson, thought the idea disastrously naive. As a result of Simpson's objections, the BMA's secretary, Dr Havard, went to Ash's headquarters in London's Mortimer Street, where the two men met for the first time and discussed their differences. Dr Havard clearly accepted the criticisms, because shortly afterwards the leaflet proposal was quietly dropped, but it was at that meeting that Simpson first told the BMA that he would welcome a greater involvement by them in the smoking issue.

It was these tentative and unsuccessful attempts by the BMA to enter the anti-smoking campaign which eventually persuaded Pamela Taylor, the BMA's press officer and parliamentary lobbyist, that the time had come to stop nibbling away at the edges of the issue. What was now required was an all-out attack on the tobacco industry. Hitherto she had always rejected such an approach because she believed it would fail. Now with the British cigarette market in decline, public opinion perceptibly changing and BMA leaders more receptive to the idea of campaigning, she thought the balance was swinging in favour of a major campaign.

Having worked in the BMA's Press and Information Division for seven years, Pamela Taylor had gained considerable experience in the art of campaigning and parliamentary lobbying, and the BMA itself had won some notable battles. It was in the forefront of the campaign for drink and driving legislation, which was acknowledged by the Minister of Transport to have been based on the BMA's recommendations. In 1981 the BMA was finally successful in securing legislation on the compulsory wearing of seat belts, although this campaign took almost 10 years to achieve its aims. In 1983 the Association mounted a massive lobbying campaign against the Government's Police and Criminal Evidence Bill to protect the confidentiality of doctors' medical records, and with the organized support of thousands of doctors the Association eventually persuaded the Government to think again. It also lobbied the Government successfully after the Data Protection Bill, which emerged shortly afterwards and which represented a similar threat to the confidentiality of medical records. However, taking on the highly

skilled and immensely wealthy tobacco industry would be very different. Not only were the companies able to draw on vast financial
resources, but their support in Parliament was considerable. One
estimate in 1981 by Mike Daube,[3] a former director of ASH, was that
the industry could count on the support of around 100 MPs, a combi-
nation of those representing constituencies containing tobacco factories and those with financial links with the tobacco or advertising industries.

So Pamela Taylor knew that if the BMA was to launch a concerted
campaign, it would have to be meticulously prepared. In early 1984
she began her research. She first had to discover who else was in
the field—an indication of the BMA's own blatant lack of knowledge
about the campaigning situation. She also talked to numerous MPs
and found to her dismay that the message of the tobacco industry was
deeply ingrained. Whenever the subject of smoking came up at
Westminster, open discussion suddenly gave way to automatic
responses. She then broached the matter informally with colleagues
inside the BMA, with Dr John Dawson, in charge of the Association's
Professional and Scientific section, and with Tim Albert, newly
appointed editor of the Association's monthly publication *BMA News
Review*. Both had no doubt that a campaign should be mounted and
they were to become key figures in the months ahead.

Perhaps the greatest fillip came when representatives of the BMA's
junior doctors discovered in the spring of 1984 that BMA Services, a
newly formed company run jointly by the BMA and the brokers Jardine
Glanvill, were recommending doctors to invest in a package of
unit trusts which included tobacco shares. This caused a considerable
furore. The first attempt by the young doctors to force BMAS to
exclude tobacco investments from its portfolio failed when in April
the Junior Members' Forum, the year's main conference for junior
doctors, rejected their plea at its meeting in Oxford by just one vote.
The publicity which this attracted focused even more attention on the
issue and when the junior doctors raised the matter again at the BMA's
annual representative meeting in Manchester in July, they were more
successful. Led by an eloquent newcomer to annual meetings, Dr
Gabriel Scally, a young community medicine trainee from Belfast, the
juniors managed to persuade the meeting to overturn the advice from
the BMA establishment and to vote for severing all links with unit
trusts investing in tobacco companies. It was this vote, 169 to 99,
demonstrating quite clearly the strength of feeling among doctors'
representatives, that convinced Pamela Taylor she had picked the
right time to press for a major campaign. Consequently, when she

formally approached BMA secretary, Dr John Havard, after the Manchester meeting to talk about the possibility of an open ended campaign, she found him totally receptive.

Dr Havard explained: 'This was the sort of thing a professional association like ours ought to be doing. We have had to fight in the past against reaction to get things like medical registration in 1858 and drink–driving legislation. All the time we have been campaigning, but far more actively recently, in favour of public health measures. It is one of the things that distinguish us from an industrial union—the work we have done, on crash helmets, on drinking and driving and seat belts has probably led directly to the redundancy of our members. Can you see an industrial union behaving like that?'

The BMA anti-smoking campaign was an idea whose time had clearly come, but having secured official approval from Dr Havard and the chief officers of the Association, the next, and perhaps more difficult, task was to open talks with ASH. Relations between the two organizations had not been good since ASH effectively torpedoed the BMA's anti-smoking leaflet two years earlier. John Dawson in particular was still smarting from David Simpson's criticism of the leaflet, which was Dawson's particular brainchild. There was also little communication between the two organizations despite the fact that their aims on smoking were so similar. Neither Pamela Taylor nor John Dawson had ever met ASH's director, David Simpson, although he was known as one of the country's leading professional campaigners, and neither side knew much about the other's organization.

Consequently, when the BMA contacted ASH to suggest a meeting at the end of August 1984 it was a crucial moment. Without ASH's full support and cooperation a major campaign by the BMA would be considerably weakened. The reason was quite clear. ASH was the country's leading campaigner in this field. It had been in existence since 1971 when it was established under the auspices of the Royal College of Physicians following the RCP's second report *Smoking and Health Now*. Since then it had become the most vociferous and experienced of the tobacco industry's opponents. Although it lacked the BMA's prestige and infrastructure, it alone had the knowledge and expertise which would be crucial to the BMA if it wanted to take on the tobacco companies.

When Pamela Taylor and John Dawson went to ASH to meet David Simpson and his deputy Patti White, they explained that they were latecomers in the anti-smoking field and that they wanted to organize a campaign which would not cut across the work of ASH and would seek to prevent the industry from persuading young people to take up smoking. Simpson was delighted. It was the biggest development that had happened during his six years at ASH. 'It was like the Americans entering the Second World War', he said.

While Simpson had to make do with a work force of three full time officials and five support staff housed in cramped third-floor London offices, the BMA was a vast organization, the medical profession's trade union and one of the most highly organized professional bodies in the country. It had recently set up a highly efficient and highly trained network of regional staff with well organized information links, and at its London headquarters had both a press office and a parliamentary unit. It also boasted an impressive track record of promoting health measures against determined opposition. Whereas the Association's membership had declined during the 1960s and early 1970s the changes introduced in the 1980s had led to a rapid increase in membership from 47 per cent of the active profession in 1977 to 72 per cent, a clear indication of support.

More important was the realization at that August meeting that the BMA was uniquely placed to spearhead an anti-smoking campaign, because it was not inhibited by having to rely on the Government for its money either directly or indirectly. ASH, on the other hand, depended on the Government for 90 per cent of its income in the form of an annual grant from the Department of Health and Social Security, which in 1984/5 amounted to £130,000. Consequently, it felt itself to some extent constrained in what it could say or do.

From that first meeting, ASH and the BMA were to develop a close and harmonious relationship which was to underpin the coming campaign. However, for diplomatic reasons it was agreed from the outset that ASH should adopt a deliberately low profile throughout the campaign, advising behind the scenes rather than being seen to sit publicly alongside the BMA. It was accepted on both sides that the BMA's influential and traditional role as the medical adviser to the nation should not be weakened in any way by being seen to be too closely aligned to a well-known pressure group.

A series of informal meetings followed over the next six weeks at which Pamela Taylor and John Dawson learned from ASH everything they could about campaigning against the tobacco industry. 'In the early meetings', said Simpson, 'we were asking things like how the BMA was structured and we were telling them about sports and arts sponsorship and how the tobacco industry had diversified into other goods and services, like adventure holidays'. The BMA employed a research student two days a week to prepare the groundwork for a campaign. By now the Association had a clear idea of the sort of campaign it wanted to mount. Its aim was a full scale Tobacco Act to ban advertising and sponsorship and it wanted to do this by dividing its campaign between the two issues. Simpson was able to advise the BMA on the key people to involve in the campaign, in particular representatives from the Health Education Council. The HEC had a budget of £2½ million to spend on anti-smoking activities, but because it was a Government-appointed and Government-funded body it could not be seen to be involved directly in lobbying.

However, it was happy to put its experience at the BMA's disposal and it went on to play a rather larger part in events than was ever publicly recognized. John Hitchins, head of public affairs at the HEC, and Linda Seymour, also from the council and formerly of ASH, were closely involved in assisting the BMA. Other individuals from other organizations were also recruited and from these names was to emerge a group of people who were to coordinate Britain's anti-smoking activities in a way that had not been attempted before.

REFERENCES

1. DHSS press release, 14 September, 1983.
2. 'UK Companies, Products and the Sports They Sponsor'. *Sportscan*.
3. *The Times*, 17 November 1981.

LESSONS FOR CAMPAIGNERS

Base your campaign on your organization's policies

Before going public check your organization's views in key areas (such as smoking and children) and the need for legislation. Organizations with no specific policies, or no mechanism for their formal creation, may want to draw up a list of points for general agreement.

Research thoroughly all sides of the argument before going public

Know your side of the story and what the opposition is likely to say. Study the scientific case: any health, economic, demographic statistics and any market analysis (who buys? where? when? etc.) you can find. Study the interests and voting patterns of MPs. Document the legal position thoroughly.

Identify your allies and keep them informed

Find out who are your friends. Contact other campaigning organizations before your launch. They will have advice to pass on, based on their experience. It is easy to start promoting ideas which others have tried and rejected. Talk to your friends and keep in regular contact.

Coordinate all activities

The aim should be to add impact and avoid conflicts. Some groups and organizations are better equipped than others to campaign on particular aspects of the issue, so don't get in their way. Avoid duplication of effort; it dilutes scarce resources and can lead to conflicting or confusing statements.

Keep your interested MPs briefed on all relevant developments

A procedure should be set up to keep informed any MPs involved in planning parliamentary activity. They will be able to table parliamentary questions at short notice in order to obtain information or make a point. They will also be able to influence the arguments of other MPs and even ministers, and should refer to the campaign's policies whenever they can.

THE LAUNCH

The press conference which launched the BMA's campaign was held on the morning of Tuesday 16 October 1984 at BMA House in London's Tavistock Square. The venue was the Princes Room, an elegant high ceilinged setting which had been festooned for the occasion with a profusion of colourful cigarette posters, leaflets and magazine advertisements showing the range of events sponsored by the tobacco companies. There were mannequins on display, their clothes bedecked with tobacco company logos, huge blown-up photographs of cigarette promotions showing children picking up advertising forms and a continuous slide show of photographs of shop window displays.

'The BMA believes all the promotional material in this room should be made illegal', said BMA secretary Dr John Havard in his opening statement to the gathering of journalists. 'You have available a list of the material we have gathered. This is just a fraction of the glossy and expensive material the tobacco industry pumps out daily and it is impossible for any of us, children, young people and adults, to avoid it. The tobacco industry spends millions of pounds employing advertising, public relations and promotional experts to help it promote a product we know—and they should know—is directly responsible for disease, illness and death.

'Advertising, sports and arts sponsorship, competitions, clothes bearing brand names and holidays are all part of the industry's attempt to fool their consumers into believing smoking is glamorous, healthy and desirable. These same consumers are our patients, and we know the truth—that smoking causes appalling illness and so many unnecessary deaths that the figure of 100,000 premature deaths a year is almost beyond comprehension.

'Tobacco companies are responsible for a massive cover-up exercise carried out worldwide by an industry which callously ignores the medical facts. They are determined, through their highly sophisticated promotional activities, to persuade millions of people to ignore the appalling health hazards, lulling them into a false sense of security by associating their products with healthy activities.

'It has to stop. And we intend to push to outlaw tobacco advertising and tobacco sponsorship. Every day we delay in banning the promotional activities of this industry, another 274 premature deaths occur. The tobacco industry is, of course, interested in market shares and profits, and successive Governments have not hesitated to use the industry's money in sponsorship of sports and the arts. Doctors are in a unique position to speak out for the rights of the individual. As doctors, we must all now speak out or be guilty of collusion.

'We will be contacting the BBC and IBA regarding tobacco sponsorship of televised events and the gratuitous smoking on television programmes. Television companies know they have a special responsibility to discourage young people from taking up smoking.

'We will tell the Government that the Health Promotion Research Trust should be closed down. The Trust was set up with tobacco industry money to carry out medical research into just about anything except the deaths and disease caused by smoking. This money should be channelled into the Medical Research Council, which has recently suffered cuts, where it can be allocated free from direction by the tobacco industry.

'We will be seeking a meeting with the Association of Chief Police Officers in an attempt to obtain police cooperation in stopping the scandalous sale of cigarettes to children. We will also be pushing to raise the legal age for buying tobacco products from 16 to 18 years old.

'We will also be requesting meetings with editors of women's magazines. Far more girls and young women are smoking—we believe this is because the tobacco companies have geared their products to attract women. A graph is available for your information. Yet the pages of women's magazines are packed with glossy advertisements for cigarettes while the articles on health rarely feature the dangers of smoking. We hope magazines will campaign with us, putting the health of their readers before tobacco advertising income.

'Throughout the coming months, the BMA will build up a special register of doctors who are willing to campaign locally. These doctors, together with our Honorary Officers in all areas, will be provided with the information they will need to carry forward the campaign locally.

'The BMA will urge individual doctors to speak out. In *BMA News Review* we give an example of a letter doctors can send to their MPs each time a patient dies prematurely from smoking.

'The BMA will act to protect young people from the tobacco industry's pressures, and we will help individual smokers fight to get the tobacco industry off their backs.

'I have written to the Secretary of State asking for the introduction of legislation to control tobacco advertising and sponsorship, and to introduce realistic health warnings.'

Then Dr John Dawson, Head of the BMA's Professional Division, followed with a statement giving the reasons for the campaign.

'We all know tobacco is a killer. Doctors know it, the public knows it and the tobacco industry ought to know it. Year after year, doctors at the BMA's Annual Representative Meeting have called for legal controls, but instead we have voluntary agreements, cosily agreed between successive Governments and the manufacturers. These agreements—as you can see—are a sick joke.

'That is why the BMA has decided to campaign against the industry's promotional activities.

'*BMA News Review* has been designed as a special campaign guide for doctors. Its purpose is to give doctors around the country the information they need to take on the tobacco industry's promotions.

'We have written to the Secretary of State, asking that legislation be introduced to ban all advertising, including advertisements in shops, all sponsorship and all the other promotional activities the industry creates to induce people to smoke and to keep on smoking. We also want realistic health warnings.

'The current health warning is a scandal. Tucked away on the side of the packet is "Cigarettes can seriously damage your health". Those cigarettes can kill people. The BMA wants to see health warnings on the front of packets linking the brand name with the deaths they cause from cancer and other diseases. These health warnings would tell the truth and the BMA believes the DHSS has a responsibility for enforcing this. Photographs of the health warning we wish to see are available.

'It is not our aim to take cigarettes away from old people who are dependent on them. This is not a campaign against the individual smoker—it is a campaign against the tobacco industry. We must help people to resist the pressures to start smoking. And that means protecting children. Because it's kids who start smoking, rarely ever adults.

'The BMA aims to cut through the millions of pounds spent by the tobacco industry to disguise what their products really are. They are trying to buy an acceptable face for a product in a way in which we say should be made illegal.

'We have begun to lobby MPs and Lords. If the Government does not have time to introduce a bill this session, we will sponsor a Private Member's Bill.

'Individuals' rights must be fought for. A child growing up in this country has a right to breathe air which is not polluted by tobacco smoke—it has been estimated that as many as 1000 non-smokers a year die from breathing other people's tobacco smoke while still more suffer unnecessary illnesses. Equally, a child has the right to grow up in a society free from the undue pressure from an industry determined to persuade him or her to start using a product carrying a 25 per cent risk of premature death. Research confirms our worst fears—that school children know the names of, and prefer to smoke, cigarette brands associated with televised sports sponsorship.

'A young adult has the right of free choice whether to smoke or not, but that right to choose does not exist in this country. A young adult cannot pick up a magazine, read a newspaper, watch the television or walk in the street without being bombarded by the tobacco industry. That is not freedom of choice, it is coercion.

'We all know that smoking can kill. The statistics show that 100,000 premature deaths each year are caused by smoking. That is 15–20 per cent of all deaths in this country. Cigarettes cause lung cancer, chronic bronchitis, emphysema and coronary heart disease, which are all killers. And we know 40 per cent of heavy smokers die before retiring age—this is compared with 15 per cent of non-smokers.

'It has been estimated that out of 1000 young men who smoke in this country, one will be murdered, six will die in a road accident and 250 will die prematurely as a result of smoking. The figures are a national disgrace.

'Quite rightly, the Government is trying to control heroin addiction—we now need legal controls to prevent young people from becoming nicotine addicts. And it is not just the nicotine—there are over 2000 other chemical agents in a cigarette, many of which initiate and promote cancer. If a drug is found to cause death or disability through adverse reactions, it is either banned or put under strict control. That is what society expects. Yet there are no legal controls on the promotion of cigarettes. The BMA believes this must be changed.'

The press conference lasted little more than an hour, although it had taken months to prepare. Dr Havard and Dr Dawson had spent countless hours being briefed and rehearsed in all aspects of their anti-smoking argument. Rarely had the BMA taken so much time on background preparation, but it was essential. The apparent simplicity of the subject, smoking and its proven dangers, was in marked contrast to the complexity of the public relations exercise needed to put it across. 'What should have been a simple subject because we are right, was in fact the most complex PR subject I have ever encountered', said Pamela Taylor.

The press conference, however, was only one leg of the launch. Selected MPs were written to and informed about the campaign, but for doctors themselves the focal point of the launch was a special edition of *BMA News Review* published to coincide with the launch day and containing practical advice to the profession on how to combat the activities of the tobacco industry. If Dr Havard had sounded the battle cry, *BMA News Review*, circulating to 73,000 doctors in the United Kingdom, was to provide the ammunition which doctors would need to fight the battle. Tim Albert, who had only recently taken over as editor, had revitalised *News Review* and was eager to involve the publication in a campaigning issue of this nature. The October edition was almost entirely devoted to smoking with a striking front cover, the work of art editor Chris Hopkins, picturing a clear blue sky above the French Alps under the logo entitled 'Breathe'. This was to become a recurring symbol in the months ahead. 'What we wanted to do was create a more positive idea', said Albert, 'rather than the usual box of dog ends and ash trays of cigarette butts. That is really only educating people to the drawbacks. We wanted to educate them to the benefits of not smoking'.

The October edition of the magazine was increased in size and contained a shortened version of the maiden speech delivered in the House of Lords four months earlier by the Duke of Gloucester, patron of ASH; an article by BBC journalist Peter Taylor, author of *The Smoke Ring*, the recently published exposé of the way the tobacco industry was protected by powerful vested interests; and a study of the scientific aspects of smoking by the BMA's president, Sir Douglas Black. However, for individual doctors, perhaps the most useful article was the one by medical journalist Olivia Timbs detailing the variety of initiatives available to them to try and change the climate of local opinion. She quoted Dr Noel Olsen, district medical officer for Hampstead in north London, saying 'If one doctor sends a letter to his MP he must be a crank. If two doctors send letters it looks like a conspiracy and they are writing on behalf of a pressure group. If three or more doctors write, that's public opinion'.

It was this article which encouraged doctors to write to their MPs whenever one of their patients died of a smoking-related disease, an idea first proposed by former ASH director, Mike Daube. Reproduced in *News Review* was a letter doctors could write to MPs. There was also a suggestion that doctors could put pressure on their local councils to ban tobacco advertising on council-owned hoardings or write to local restaurants, pubs, sports clubs, banks and cinemas outlining the rights of non-smokers to breathe clean air. Finally, at the back of *News Review* was a coupon for doctors to fill in if they were willing to be included on a new BMA register of people prepared actively to campaign against smoking.

The hope was that 50 to 100 doctors might eventually register. The returns, however, were to exceed all expectations.

LESSONS FOR CAMPAIGNERS

Develop simple ideas that will capture the public imagination

It is important to attract attention from the media and the public. They will not understand the issues as well as you, so think of simple images they can easily identify. Think of the World Wildlife Fund panda, the chain of humans holding hands at Greenham Common, the CND symbol, the BUGA-UP poster campaign. The tobacco industry uses such simple ideas; so must campaigners.

Develop your own style and language

Work out an appropriate public profile; for example, anti-Government or learned/scientific. Adopt an appropriate language. Never use the phrases which the tobacco industry and its supporters use.

Be flexible

You must be able to respond to the unexpected and make it difficult for an unexpected opposition ploy to 'unseat' you. Few campaigners have the resources to match the opposition so stay in front and do not be 'wrong footed'. Always try to have one or two contingency plans so that you can change direction quickly if you have to. Remember the opposition may do something unpredicted, and you may have to mount a sudden press conference to respond.

Try to anticipate the opposition, but do not be complacent

This is difficult—even with moles, but trying to understand what the opposition thinks or is planning will help you to decide on your tactics. Don't bank on being correct, but try to get as much information as you can, and use your judgement carefully.

Use all the media

They are one of your best assets, so spend time and effort learning how to serve journalists and preparing useful briefs. Don't expect reporters to write up any press release, or editors to give it space, just because the cause is worthy. Link your story to some context (or 'peg', as journalists call it) which will make your story interesting and topical. For example, don't mention your plan for more tax on cigarettes in the summer recess but wait until a month before the budget. Release your comment about alcohol and road traffic accidents on the day that the Minister of Transport releases the annual road death figures. Link your attack on sports sponsorship by tobacco companies to a major sponsored tournament. Pegs alone are not enough; there must be a story. That Big Ben strikes twelve at midnight again isn't a story, but it is if it strikes thirteen! Present the story so that a journalist can use it; there's an art to writing a good press release, but it can be learned quickly.

Develop campaign images through 'positive' logos

Visual images are vital. A logo (a symbol which is used on all correspondence, publications, etc.) is useful to illustrate the message of the campaign and also to act as a flag. Logos should be simple to understand and positive. Don't use negative ideas, such as ashtrays brimming with cigarettes but concentrate on more positige images such as breathing clean air. One warning: engage the services of a professional designer; the work of an amateur tends to look amateurish—and gives the campaign a high-profile bad image.

Know your friends and foes in Commons and Lords

Research the voting patterns and activities of MPs and Lords by looking up previous debates; who signed early day motions; who asked parliamentary questions; and who said what to the press. Compile lists of obvious supporters and opponents.

Cooperate with any house magazine

House magazines can help with the launch, and after that to report how the campaign is developing, and as another way of initiating stories. A launch issue should contain background material, articles from 'personalities' that can be picked up by the press, and information for readers (members of your organization) on how they can help. Cut-out forms can be used to build up a central register of supporters; readers are committed once they have sent these off. Use your logo freely. Link publication in with press conferences.

Know parliamentary procedures

You must be able to use parliamentary procedures fully and know, for example, the dates for second readings, the background reading to Early Day Motions, the various types of Parliamentary Questions and debates. These procedures can then be used to full advantage.

Cultivate the MPs who support you

From your lists of those MPs and Lords who support you, choose a couple from each House to help plan activities. They should be known to be active on the issue.

Involve your members

Remember to involve members, supporters or volunteers so that they become part of the campaign. Keep them informed and involved, so they can build on their initial efforts, and encourage them to feed back information for central coordination and action. House magazines and newsletters can help keep up momentum.

Make sure the Government's position is made public

The campaign is necessary because Government has not acted on the issue, and it is useful to have on record, for example, its refusal to introduce legislation to control tobacco advertising and sponsorship and realistic health warnings. Write to the Secretary of State urging legislation and publish his answer.

THE BLACK-EDGED CARDS

The campaign launch attracted considerable media attention both on television and in the national and provincial press. 'Doctors call for end to all advertising by tobacco companies' was the headline in *The Times*, 'Tobacco promotion ban sought' in the *Financial Times* and 'Doctors' War on Smoking' in the *Daily Star*. With the publicity came the criticism. The Tobacco Advisory Council, the mouthpiece of the industry, was widely quoted[1] on the morning after the press conference as stating that the BMA had never produced any evidence that a ban on sponsorship or advertising would reduce either overall consumption or the number of people, including young people, deciding to start smoking. The pro-smoking group FOREST pointed out[2] that tobacco advertising was banned in Communist countries and yet consumption there was still increasing.

A letter in the *Daily Telegraph*[3] from Sir Edward Tuckwell, former surgeon to the Queen, said: 'If you attend any medical congress, smoking may be banned in the auditorium, but outside many, many doctors will be polluting the air and other people's lungs. Unless the majority of doctors give up smoking I feel that the BMA is not speaking for the profession, but for a rather rarer group'. Less than 15 per cent of doctors still smoke.

Tobacco shares fell slightly in the aftermath of the launch, recovering later, but the announcement which was to cause the greatest stir as a result of the press conference was something which the BMA had neither intended nor prepared for. Buried in two of the following day's newspaper reports[4] of the press conference was the news that the BMA was printing thousands of black-edged postcards to be distributed to doctors to send to MPs when a patient of theirs died from smoking. The cards would read: 'I wish to inform you that one of your constituents, who was a patient of mine, has died. I am writing to tell you this because his/her death was premature and was caused by smoking'.

The proposal, however, was not among the ideas in the *BMA News Review*, nor was it contained in the opening statements from Dr Havard and Dr Dawson or in the replies to the questions that followed. This was because, quite simply, it was a spur of the moment idea which emerged immediately after the press conference during a conversation between Dr Dawson and a journalist. Having emerged, the idea was put into effect immediately, which was why two of the following morning's newspapers were reporting that the BMA was already printing thousands of the black-edged cards.

The incident illustrated what was to become an essential ingredient of the campaign—its flexibility. Over the coming months, decisions were to be taken by a few key people, by Dr John Havard taking ultimate responsibility with Pamela Taylor and Dr John Dawson, but they were not determining BMA policy. They were simply executing the policy as laid down by resolutions passed at successive annual representative meetings of the BMA. There were, of course, times when matters had to be referred to the chief officers of the Association or brought before its Board of Science and Education. It was also important to keep the BMA's Council informed of what was happening, but this was a body of 60 members which met only five times a year to administer affairs between the BMA's annual meetings. It could not act as a swift decision-making body. The tobacco campaign was essentially an executive management exercise which avoided all the time-consuming drawbacks of committee decision making while being careful to keep strictly within the BMA's existing policies. It thus succeeded in retaining sufficient flexibility to plan and execute as it went along.

The black-edged cards were the product of just such flexibility. Within two weeks of the 'spur of the moment' idea, the BMA's Professional Relations Unit was circulating to doctors the news that the cards had been produced, local BMA offices had initial supplies and thousands more were being run. Posters advertising the cards went to BMA notice boards throughout the country and secretaries of BMA divisions were asked to publicise them. Arrangements were made to include a leaflet about the campaign with the subscription renewal notices going to every member in the next few weeks and they were sent to every new member joining the Association in the following months. In its letter it said: 'The BMA is urging doctors to write to the MPs of any patients who die through a smoking-induced disease. Black-edged postcards have been produced for this purpose. If only a proportion of the deaths are reported in this way, it will have a major impact and bring home to MPs the extent of the problem. Please put your name and address or surgery stamp on the card. It is important to include this information on each occasion to show that the cards are authentic and, of course, MPs may wish to reply. There is a different serial number on each postcard which may be used for reference purposes. You may wish to make a note of the number in the patient's record.

'You will need to write the name of the patient's MP on the front of the card. If you do not know the constituency or the name, telephone the electoral registration officer at the local town hall, who will be able to identify the relevant constituency easily. In the case of hospital doctors, whose patients' homes may not be in the same area as the hospital, provided they have the full address of the patient, the House of Commons information office says it will always be able to help.

'The wording on the card refers to "a patient of mine"; we hope that consultants and junior doctors will be able to come to a suitable arrangement so that a card may be sent each time a patient dies from a smoking-related disease.

'Further supplies of the postcard are available from local BMA offices. Thank you for your assistance'.

This was important as it pre-empted later criticisms that the doctor was breaking confidentiality.

Doctors were asked to tick one of four boxes alongside 'lung cancer', 'chronic obstructive lung disease', 'coronary heart disease' and 'other tobacco-related cancer or vascular disease'. The BMA estimated that if every doctor were to send in details of each patient who died through smoking, 270 black-edged cards would arrive each day at the House of Commons. 'Even if a tenth of this, 27 cards a day, were sent to the Commons', said Dr Dawson, 'that is still a steady trickle of correspondence which would be instantly identifiable. We knew this would stimulate a lot of controversy. But we decided at the time that we should make a conscious effort to be hard about this'.

The campaign was now well under way. Parliamentary Bills were being drafted and a series of parliamentary questions were to be tabled with three aims—to obtain information needed later in the campaign, to stimulate parliamentary awareness and to provide information for press comment. Two MPs, Roger Sims (Con., Chislehurst) and Laurie Pavitt (Lab., Brent South) had tabled an early day motion in the House of Commons urging the Government 'to take steps to ensure that children grow up free from pressures to smoke, by phasing out the promotional activities of the tobacco companies and enforcing the law relating to the sale of cigarettes to children under 16 years of age, in view of the established evidence and the mounting concern of the medical profession that smoking-induced diseases are the single most important cause of avoidable death in the United Kingdom'.

Doctors and others were being urged to write to their MPs asking them to sign the motion or state their reasons for refusing to sign. Early day motions—so-called because those MPs signing them were effectively urging the Government to find an early day to debate the topic—rarely if ever led to debate or early action.

However, as effective propaganda they were invaluable, not only to air a particular issue but also to give organizations such as the BMA an excuse for approaching MPs for support. This enabled them to identify sympathetic MPs with whom further contact could be made and conversely to identify hostile MPs.

Occasionally, MPs moved from one camp to the other. Conservative MP Roger Sims was one such example. At the time of the BMA's campaign against the Government on the Police and Criminal Evidence Bill in 1983, the Minister it had to deal with was the Home Secretary, William Whitelaw. His parliamentary private secretary at the time and the man responsible for liaising between the two sides was Roger Sims. As the BMA's campaign intensified, relations between the doctors and the Government became distinctly strained. A year later when Pamela Taylor began canvassing parliamentary support on the tobacco campaign, she first of all sought out the chairman of the all-Party group for action on smoking and health and discovered to her dismay that it was Roger Sims. At first, relations between the two were not easy and the BMA had to do some quick fence mending, but on the smoking issue Sims was quite clearly on the same side, having sponsored a Bill for non-smokers as long ago as 1977, and eventually a rapport developed and Sims became one of the BMA's staunchest allies. He had first taken an interest in smoking when he was a member of the All-party Commons Social Services committee in 1974/5 which reported on preventive medicine. 'I thought the evidence we had then was overwhelming as to the harm done by smoking and the amount of smoking-related disease there was and of course its effect on both the cost of the health service, not to mention the human misery'. However, he said he was not a zealot on the issue. 'I am not myself a smoker, but I have members of my own family who smoke and I realize that to a lot of people it does mean a great deal. So the idea of banning smoking is simply impracticable'. He also said that there was an obligation on the Government to ensure that the knowledge there was about the harmful effect of smoking was disseminated as widely as possible so that moves could be made towards the eventual abolition of tobacco promotion.

Labour MP Laurie Pavitt had been involved in the issue for even longer, ever since he introduced his first anti-smoking—or as he prefers to call it 'pro-health'—Bill in 1966. He described the BMA's campaign as 'the biggest step forward we have had'. He said: 'During the period since the 1960s the medical profession has been able to express itself mainly through the Royal College of Physicians, but they did not have clout. The BMA has clout. It is probably the most effective lobby in the House of Commons other than the National Farmers Union. In the past we have had plenty of brains. Now we have plenty of muscle'.

While sympathetic MPs were being sought out to support the

campaign, the BMA made its first direct approach to Ministers. Three weeks after the campaign launch, a senior BMA deputation went to the Department of Health and Social Security to meet Ministers. Led by Dr John Marks, a practising general practitioner and chairman of the BMA Council, the deputation consisted of Dr John Havard, secretary of the Association, and the chairmen of the BMA's four main professional committees representing the whole medical profession—for the consultants Dr Maurice Burrows of the central committee for hospital medical services, for GPs Dr Michael Wilson of the general medical services committee, for junior hospital doctors Dr Robert Hangartner and for community doctors Dr David Miles.

On the Government's side were Norman Fowler, Secretary of State for Social Services, Kenneth Clarke, the Minister of State for Health, John Patten, Parliamentary Under Secretary of State, and Dr Donald Acheson, the Chief Medical Officer.

The outcome of the meeting from the BMA's point of view was not very fruitful. Norman Fowler listened to the Association's views on sports sponsorship and quite rightly replied that this was a matter not for him but for the Sports Minister and the Department of the Environment. However, what he and his Ministerial colleagues did say gave the BMA no cause for thinking that they were ready to do anything to curb the activities of the tobacco companies, even though only the previous week John Patten had spoken at the launch of the Health Education Council's 'Pacesetters Don't Smoke' campaign aimed at persuading young people not to smoke. Kenneth Clarke, whose parliamentary constituency of Rushcliffe in Nottingham was the home of the tobacco company John Player, appeared totally unmoved by what he heard. However, Dr Marks said afterwards: 'Mr Fowler was very sympathetic to the idea of a smoking campaign, though it was a disappointing meeting in so far as he did not have the power to do anything'.

It was, however, a necessary meeting for the BMA to enable it at the start of the campaign to assess ministerial opinion. In the weeks and months to come, as the campaign developed, there were indications that Ministers were beginning to come under some pressure as a result of the campaign. The word from the DHSS was that officials wished the BMA would stop agitating so much. There were also reports that health ministers were considering their own anti-smoking campaign in response to the BMA, but had been warned by their specialist advisers that this would simply draw attention to smoking and encourage more youngsters to smoke.

Already, after only a few weeks of the campaign, the BMA could point with some success to an upsurge of anti-tobacco stories appearing in the press and to a general anti-smoking climate beginning to permeate the media.

REFERENCES

1. *The Guardian, Financial Times, Sheffield Morning Telegraph*, 17 October 1984.
2. *Glasgow Herald*, 17 October 1984.
3. *Daily Telegraph*, 22 October 1984.
4. *The Times, Daily Telegraph*, 17 October 1984.

LESSONS FOR CAMPAIGNERS

Tell your members what you are doing and involve other specialist services within your organization

Work with your colleagues. There may be in-house experts in communications, design, law and research. Ask for their advice and give them time and room to help, wherever possible, on their terms. Small organizations and groups should work together to exploit existing expertise. Don't alienate colleagues by forgetting to keep them informed.

Don't underestimate constituents' responses to MPs

Although the organization at national level would be in touch with MPs, local constituents (i.e. voters) carry a great deal of weight. They should comment on developments in the campaign and on any public statements made by the MP. Meet the MP personally. These communications should be relevant to the MP's constituency.

Plan carefully, but be aware of how unexpected events have contributed to past successes

Appreciate the value of the unexpected, like Princess Margaret's doctors advising her against smoking, a leading heart transplant surgeon recommending surgery for prevention, the Minister of Health giving the Health Education Council an extra £500,000 to spend on a cigarette advertising campaign in just six months, or the black-edged cards, which caught the media's attention and led the BMA to implement them immediately.

Use parliamentary questions and early day motions

PQs are tabled because they stimulate parliamentary awareness, and are a way of getting information from civil servants. It is useful to have the up-to-date statistics for such things as writing letters and preparing briefing documents. You can time them for answering on a specific day, and they can then be used as a 'peg' for publicity. Early day motions are not normally debated, but are a useful method of gauging the views of MPs: local MPs' views can be canvassed and the MPs initiating the motion can 'lobby' their colleagues while in the House use the responses to update your MPs' lists. The more MPs who sign the early day motion the better, because it shows the weight of feeling in the house. If there are more than 100 signatories, the motion may be debated.

Be sensitive to the development of momentum of your campaign

Do not lose momentum, but equally do not burn yourself out. First, build up interest and support, taking care to bring your supporters with you. Building up momentum steadily will help you to present each new advance as a victory. This will let the media and others see that you are making progress. Nothing can be worse than starting off with a bang followed by 24 months of silence while you diligently plan phase II, but meanwhile slip from the memory of both public and media.

Identify some 'big guns' and hold them in reserve

These can be deployed to increase momentum or counter an unexpected move by the opposition. If you have time when nothing much happens (or everything goes wrong) bring out some eminent figure, clever stunt or scandalous data.

INFLUENCING THE YOUNG

With the campaign now in its third month, reaction was still highly encouraging. 'It seems to have caught the imagination of doctors and the public', said Pamela Taylor. 'Doctors have been ringing in numbers we have never known before, saying that they are happy to help in any way'.[1] Public response had also been favourable and letters of inquiry had come in from such diverse interested bodies as the Department of Health in Dublin, the Australian Medical Association and the Chairman of the British Airports Authority.

However, from one quarter there was comparative silence. The tobacco industry's voice had been distinctly muted. After its initial response to the campaign launch denying any link between advertising and young people starting to smoke, the industry had lapsed into silence only to attempt to reappear later on in the campaign. One reason for this was that the tobacco companies were clearly hoping they could ride out the storm and wait for the campaign to go away, but the BMA had no intention of satisfying their hopes. 'We have to keep up the pressure' Dr Havard told *BMA News Review*. 'This is the main thing we have to do now'.

To achieve this the Association had planned a rolling programme to keep up the momentum in a way it had never tried to do before. December's campaign publication was a survey by Dr Frank Ledwith, research fellow in the Department of Education at the University of Manchester, showing 'beyond any reasonable doubt' how tobacco industry sports sponsorship acted as advertisements to children, so bypassing the television advertising ban. In an article published in the *Health Education Journal*, he detailed his research, the first of its kind, carried out among 880 children in five secondary schools in Greater Manchester, which found that children were most aware of the cigarette brands which were most frequently associated with sponsored sporting events on TV.

He discovered that children's television viewing of the Benson and Hedges Masters snooker championship in February 1984 was positively correlated with the proportion of children associating that brand and other brands used in TV sponsorship with sport. Following the World Snooker Championship in April and May 1984 sponsored by Embassy, which attracted 100 hours of BBC television coverage, a subsequent survey was carried out on a new sample, showing that awareness of this brand, and the proportion of children associating it with sport had increased from the first survey. This, said Dr Ledwith, demonstrated that the television sports sponsored by tobacco manufacturers acted as cigarette advertising to children and therefore circumvented the law banning cigarette advertising on television.

At a press conference on December 14 held by the BMA to announce the results of the survey, Dr John Dawson said the Association would now seek meetings with the BBC and with the Independent Broadcasting Authority to discuss ways of excluding tobacco brand names from television. He said that the BBC was probably in breach of its charter and that the independent companies were breaking the advertising ban, and he warned that the BMA would not rule out an injunction if the broadcasting authorities did not take action to rectify this.

Dr Dawson also pointed out that sponsorship by tobacco companies accounted for 10 to 15 per cent of the total funds available to sport from industry and the proportion was declining as new sponsors appeared. There was no lack of sponsorship from other sources. Athletics and swimming were cited as sports which did not accept sponsorship from the tobacco companies.

In the same week as the press conference, the December issue of BMA News Review was published with a timely seasonal warning— 'Tobacco gifts are death at Christmas'. On its front cover was a grinning skull decked out with a paper hat and surrounded by tinsel and holly and with a lighted cigarette between its teeth. The approach of Christmas had presented News Review with an ideal opportunity for a simple but effective way of building on the campaign message. 'A lot of people, including my own GP, thought the cover was too gruesome', said editor Tim Albert, 'but I thought it was right to have a cover which might offend some people'.

In an accompanying statement to the press, BMA secretary Dr John Havard said: 'The BMA this year is appealing to everyone to think twice before they buy cigarettes as presents. The tobacco industry has Christmas promotions for a substance which is known to kill 100,000 people a year prematurely. The lethal effects of cigarette smoking do not stop for the festive season. Over Christmas, registration of new cases of cancer of the lung, bronchus, pleura and trachea, mostly associated with smoking, will continue at a rate of 100 a day. Other diseases associated with smoking, such as heart disease, will also be diagnosed. Many doctors and nurses in hospitals will be caring for patients who are terminally ill as a result of their addiction to cigarettes and who will not see another Christmas.

'Particularly when you hand out those presents on the Christmas tree, the BMA entreats you not to give cigarettes to the young. Once they get addicted to smoking, it is very difficult to give it up. At Christmas time, families and friends should encourage them to live rather than die early from the effects of tobacco smoking'.

By coincidence, on the same day that the BMA's grinning skull appeared, the Chief Medical Officer at the DHSS, Dr Donald Acheson, issued his annual report 'On the State of the Public Health for the Year 1983'.[2] This showed that occasionally the Department of Health and the BMA sang the same tune. In his report Dr Acheson declared that the habit of smoking cigarettes was by far the largest avoidable hazard in Britain today and he went on: 'In 1972 the cigarette was described by one of my predecessors as "the most lethal instrument devised by man for peaceful use". Cigarette smokers are now in a minority in all social groups, but much remains to be done, both to persuade those who continue to smoke to stop, and to discourage people from starting to smoke'.

The question doctors wanted answering, however, was whether Dr Acheson's words would be backed up by Government action, but to this there was no answer.

Meanwhile the BMA announced that it was backing a Private Member's Bill in the House of Commons to ban the sponsorship of sporting events by tobacco companies. This was the first of two Bills the BMA helped to draft and although it was known that neither stood a chance of being implemented, there was the possibility that one of them would be debated in Parliament and consequently that they would attract further publicity for the campaign. As with the tabling of early day motions, a Private Member's Bill gave the BMA an opportunity to approach MPs for support and to contact the media and other interested bodies.

The first Bill, published in December, was sponsored by Conservative MP Roger Sims. Entitled the Tobacco Products (Sports Sponsorship) Bill, it consisted of four clauses and was modelled on the succession of Private Member's Bills that Labour MP Laurie Pavitt had tried and failed to introduce over the previous decade.

A
BILL
TO

Provide for a ban on sponsorship of sporting events by tobacco companies, to be achieved by progressive reduction of expenditure, and for purposes connected therewith.

1.—(1) The Secretary of State may by Order make provision for the prohibition of expenditure on sponsorship by tobacco companies of sporting events, to be achieved by a progressive reduction of expenditure, by a date to be specified in the Order being a date not later than three years from the passing of this Act.

(2) The power of the Secretary of State to make an Order under this section shall be exercisable by statutory instrument and shall be subject to annulment in pursuance of a resolution of either House of Parliament.

2.—(1) If a person contravenes an Order made under section 1 above, he shall be guilty of an offence and liable—
   (a) on conviction on indictment, to a fine;
   (b) on summary conviction, to a fine not exceeding level 4 on the standard scale and, in the case of a continuing offence, to a further fine not exceeding one tenth of level 4 on the standard scale for each day on which the offence is continued.

(2) Where an offence under this Act is committed by a body corporate or by a person purporting to act on behalf of a body corporate or an unincorporated body of persons and is proved to have been committed with the consent or approval of, or to have been facilitated by any neglect on the part of, any person, who when the offence is committed is a director, member of the committee of management or other controlling authority of the body concerned, or the manager, secretary or other officer of the body, that person shall also be deemed to have committed the offence and may be proceeded against and punished accordingly.

3. In this Act—
   "sponsorship" means the giving, or the causing to be given, of financial or other assistance to or for a person or for or in

relation to an event or activity, in consideration of the use, display, advertising or association with, or by the person or at or in connection with the event or activity (or with the name or title of the event or activity), of a tobacco product (or of the name of a brand of tobacco product);

"tobacco product" means any form of tobacco intended for smoking or chewing, including cigarettes and smoking mixtures intended as a substitute for tobacco.

4.—(1) This Act may be cited as the Tobacco Products (Sports Sponsorship) Act 1985.

(2) This Act extends to Northern Ireland.

Sponsoring the Bill with Roger Sims were three Conservative MPs, Nigel Forman (Carshalton and Wallington), Toby Jessel (Twickenham) and Sir Anthony Meyer (Clwyd NW), three Labour MPs, George Foulkes (Carrick, Cumnock and Doon Valley), Laurie Pavitt (Brent S) and Robert Sheldon (Ashton under Lyne), and a Liberal, Clement Freud (Cambridgeshire NE). The Bill was published and given its formal first reading in the Commons on December 20 and then had to join the long queue of other Private Member's Bills awaiting debate. Like most of them, however, it was to sink without trace and the BMA would have to rely on its second Bill to surface for debate. As Roger Sims explained: 'There is a very strong tobacco lobby in the Commons which will clearly try to prevent anything of this sort progressing and so the prospects of a Private Member making much progress with a Bill such as mine are pretty slim'. He also said that Bills of this sort did help to create a general awareness of smoking.

Meanwhile in the letter columns of *Pulse*, the weekly medical newspaper for GPs, the pro- and anti-smoking camps were engaged in some interesting correspondence. In an editorial in October, *Pulse* made the statement 'No-one can doubt the validity of the BMA's motives nor question the adverse effects of cigarette advertising'. This prompted Martin Mulholland, the general manager of public affairs at Gallaher, the American-owned British tobacco company, to write back saying: 'There is no evidence that cigarette advertising increases total consumption or the number of people who choose to smoke. Such a ban (on advertising) would therefore not have the effect hoped for by the BMA. On the other hand, cigarette advertising is known to influence smokers' choice of brands and provide smokers with information, for instance on tar levels. Without advertising research and development would lose their commercial purpose, because the public could not be informed of the qualities of the resulting new and modified products. For doctors to support a ban without insisting on seeing sound evidence of its likely effects will certainly invite challenges from MPs and others'.

It was now the turn of Dr John Dawson of the BMA to take up his pen. 'Is Gallaher's Martin Mulholland seriously asking us to believe cigarette advertising "provides smokers with information"?

'A nameless piece of slashed silk (Silk Cut), an underwater scene (Benson and Hedges), or a picture of a Marlboro pack, captioned "the world's best-selling cigarette" bears no reference to the truth that cigarettes cause 100,000 premature deaths every year in this country from cancer, coronary heart disease and other tobacco-related cancer or vascular disease. Mr Mulholland then asks us to accept that "there is no evidence that cigarette advertising increases total consumption". Advertisers of other products believe advertising increases sales. If cigarette advertising is unique, why would developing countries with state-organized tobacco monopolies need to advertise, other than to boost sales?

'Finally, he claims there is no evidence that cigarette advertising increases "the number of people who choose to smoke". We all know it is children, rarely ever adults, who start to smoke. What choice do our children have when they are bombarded by an industry spending millions on promotion? For years the tobacco industry lobby has had its own way. Far from fearing MPs' challenges, the BMA welcomes the opportunity of giving them the facts'.

The correspondence closed with a letter from David Simpson of ASH in which he said there was plenty of evidence that cigarette advertising increased sales, undermined health education and helped to recruit new generations of children to the smoking habit. 'It is revealing to ask why there is aggressive advertising in developing countries where one company has a monopoly. Or why, when the chips are down and the industry is threatened by an advertising ban, the cigarette pushers say in desperation that, if enacted, the ban will "destroy our business". How could that possibly be so if advertising did not affect total sales?'

David Simpson went on: 'The temerity of these people in saying that they need advertising to convey information on tar levels is even more breathtaking. Not prepared to admit their products are lethal, they coyly allude to the fact that some may be slightly less lethal than others. And since that part of smoking and health policy which covers slightly less lethal cigarettes offers a glimmer of hope of continuing sales, they desperately try to elevate the subject to a position of priority; and worse still, they use it to try to blackmail policymakers to leave advertising alone.

'If scientific opinion dictates that there should be further changes in emission levels (and there are strong signs that perhaps there should be no more) then those must be controlled by powers in the hands of health ministers, backed up by force of law. And to inform the public, what better than the Government's existing publication, the tables of tar, nicotine and carbon monoxide yields of all cigarettes on the market? The pushers know that their advertising is vital to continue recruiting children to smoking. That is why they will fight an advertising ban to the bitter end. And that is why the BMA's campaign is so very important for the health of future generations'.

REFERENCES

1. *BMA News Review*, December 1984.
2. DHSS press release, 10 December 1984.
3. *Pulse*, November 17, December 1 and 24, 1984.

LESSONS FOR CAMPAIGNERS

Use the letter columns of journals and newspapers, in particular local ones

Letter pages are among the most read pages. They also allow anybody to get into print. Use a 'peg' if you can—for example react to a story in the publication—but letters must be short (three paragraphs?). Don't try to make too many points. Phone the letters' editor to discuss the points you want to make and ask about their policy on letters. This will make your letter anonymous among the others in the sack. Type your letter in double spacing, and don't forget to put a name, address and phone number.

Cooperate with other campaigners

Help others to build a platform. There are individuals and groups with
interesting things to say but who lack the facilities to campaign publicly. Work together and pool resources. You can approach larger
organizations for help particularly with organizing press conferences.

Use Private Members' Bills

Private Member's Bills are introduced by backbench MPs rather than
the Government. They are given only a limited amount of time and
few succeed, but they are a useful vehicle for gauging support in the
House and getting publicity. If the Bill is debated, the issue will be
aired and the opposition's arguments brought out. Private Member's
Bills in the Lords normally have debate (second reading), but in the
Commons a debate can be blocked by anyone who opposes the Bill.
All-party support is important.

Don't duck politically sensitive aspects

Make sure that the final decisions on sensitive issues are taken at the
highest level of your organization—and that they will stand. Face up
to politically embarrassing aspects; internal rifts spell disaster. Make
sure that you inform those who should be told what is going on.

Cultivate all journalists whose interests and support you need

Even when you think journalists are against you, it's worth trying to
win them over. Contrary to what people think, the best way is not to
'bribe' them with hospitality, but give them good accurate information
they can use.

Do not ignore unsympathetic journalists

Try to get them on your side. The media are your most powerful
resource and good relationships with journalists are worth cultivating

and nurturing. Be as helpful to them as you can and be sympathetic to the pressures of their job (e.g. deadlines).

THE RED BOOK CONTROVERSY

It was perhaps surprising that the campaign so far had progressed relatively smoothly for the BMA. It had avoided any glaring tactical errors and any major internal dissent, but this peace and harmony was to be broken by what became known as The Red Book—*Report on Investment in the UK Tobacco Industry*.

As so often happens, the controversy which was about to break was not of the BMA's making. Towards the end of 1984, the Health Education Council informed the BMA that it had commissioned some research into who was investing in the major UK tobacco companies. However, having commissioned the research and seen its findings, the HEC realised that it was not the sort of survey it could publish, for it revealed that cancer research charities, hospitals, health authorities and leading medical institutions were among those who were investing in the tobacco industry, many of them unwittingly. The report listed 350 organizations with millions of pounds worth of shares in six major UK tobacco firms and read like a Who's Who of Britain's major organizations concerned with medicine and the sick.

The Health Education Council realized at once that the report would create a considerable stir and that the Council could not afford to be held responsible. As a Government-appointed body, the HEC was constantly aware of its limitations and this was one occasion when it decided that reticence would be politically wise. However, its director general Dr David Player still wanted to see the research published and so he approached the BMA.

The BMA was immediately sensitive to the likely repercussions of publication. The research named Royal Colleges and other eminent health organizations with whom the Association had close relations.

Some of them were involved in the very campaign on which the BMA was now embarked. Publication was bound to embarrass all of them and anger many of them. So should the BMA take the risk in publishing the facts? Although the research had been commissioned by the HEC, it had actually been carried out by David Gilbert of Social

Audit, a small, independent, non-profit making body on the left-wing fringe of the pressure-group world. What little the BMA knew of the organization it did not like. Social Audit was among the strongest advocates of reducing the NHS drugs bill by curtailing doctors' freedom to prescribe what they liked—a viewpoint strongly opposed by the BMA, which was currently engaged in a fierce dispute with the Government over its plans to introduce a limited list of drugs. As a result there was a mutual mistrust between the BMA and Social Audit which never improved.

Pamela Taylor believed the BMA had to publish the report. She commented: 'We were put in a position where we couldn't refuse, because if we had we knew the material would be published anyway. It would have become the report which the BMA would not publish and that would have meant the end of our tobacco campaign. How could we have carried on after that?' Pending Dr Havard's return from leave, arrangements were made to produce the document. Only at a later stage were the chief officers of the Association notified about what was happening and some of them were horrified. The first sight that the BMA's treasurer, Dr Tony Keable-Elliott, had of the report was in its final form only days before the date provisionally fixed for the press conference. Looking down the list of companies named in the report as investing in the tobacco industry, he saw Grand Metropolitan, in which he knew the BMA itself had shares, but because these were held through nominees, the BMA was not among the list of shareholders named in the report. It was the first time it had been realized by the BMA that Grand Met had a tobacco connection through its ownership of an American tobacco company. Dr Keable-Elliott asked for an immediate meeting of the BMA's chief officers at which he objected to publication of the booklet. He said that the BMA was in danger of appearing hypocritical in arguing against holding shares in Grand Met while, for instance, allowing doctors to carry out insurance examinations for Eagle Star, a subsidiary of BAT. The border line between the two was dangerously narrow. He said that the BMA was in the same position as other organizations in holding these shares unwittingly, and that other organizations were being treated discourteously in not being given prior notice of the fact that the report was being published.

Another of the chief officers, Mr James Kyle, chairman of the Representative Body, was also against the BMA publishing the booklet. Mr Kyle, a Scottish surgeon, was not a great supporter of the smoking campaign. His objection was to a suggestion in the booklet that comprehensive searching should be carried out of registers of shareholders in tobacco companies. This, to him, meant encouraging doctors to discover the names of other doctors with shares and putting pressure on them to sell. Mr Kyle said he found this 'peeping toms' idea repugnant. However, two other chief officers and two senior officers who attended the meeting favoured publication—the BMA's president Sir Douglas Black, the chairman of council Dr John Marks, the BMA's secretary Dr Havard and the editor of the *British Medical Journal* Dr Stephen Lock. Their enthusiasm varied however. Dr Marks, for instance, was far from happy, but took the view that once the facts had been compiled they should be released.

He was insistent that there should be no cover up. The main concern of the meeting was that the BMA's own credibility would suffer if someone else published the report and revealed that the Association had refused to do so. Social Audit had made it quite clear that if the BMA refused to publish the document, it would do so and explain why. So the chief officers decided not to object to publication. Meanwhile the BMA general fund had immediately sold its Grand Met shares. It was agreed to respect the Health Education Council's wish not to be named as having commissioned the report, even though publication was being financed by the HEC. However, this was eventually leaked to the press, with the BMA pointing the finger of suspicion for the leak at Social Audit.

There was a further problem over the wording on the front cover of the report about its attribution. Dr Keable-Elliott would have liked a form of words distancing the Association from responsibility for the document. Social Audit also wanted its name on the cover, but the BMA refused, preferring instead an acknowledgement on the inside front cover. This eventually read: 'The BMA is publishing Social Audit's document so that those who may have unwittingly invested in the tobacco industry can be so informed'. There then followed a debate about whether to give those mentioned in the report prior warning of the fact. The logistical problems of having to contact some 350 different organizations would have been considerable, but it was eventually decided against any prior notification for another reason. 'It would have smacked of blackmail', said Dr Havard. 'It would have looked as if we were forcing these organizations to sell their shares, whereas of course we didn't necessarily want them to sell. There were other means to bring pressure to bear on companies to diversify'. However, the decision not to notify simply exacerbated the sense of ill feeling which surrounded the report.

The press conference launching the document was held on Sunday, 13 January 1985 with publication embargoed until the following day.

The unusual choice of a Sunday—not a popular working day for journalists, though a good day for securing maximum coverage in the national press—was forced on the BMA when it discovered that the author of the report, David Gilbert, was about to leave the country for three months and it was necessary that he should be available for the press conference. Launching the report, Dr Havard said: 'When I saw the results of the survey, I was surprised to see what organizations were holding shares in companies concerned with the tobacco industry. I really must assume that a very high number of organizations do not realise when they hold shares in the companies that they are involved in the industry'. And he added, 'This is not a witch-hunt—we regard the shareholders we name as friends and allies in our campaign to stop sports sponsorship by the tobacco industry and the advertising of tobacco products. We are asking the shareholders to consider the ethics of holding investments and receiving profits from companies which are responsible for the single, most preventable cause of death.

There are many options shareholders can take. For instance, apart from getting rid of their tobacco share investments, they could take a more active line as shareholders to bring pressure to bear on the companies they invest in'.

As expected, the report received considerable publicity in Monday morning's national and provincial newspapers and on television. 'Cancer charities in BMA list of shareholders in tobacco firms' was the headline in *The Guardian*, 'Top Health Chiefs in Tobacco Cash Shock' in *The Daily Express* and 'Tobacco Firms' Links Exposed by BMA' in the *Western Mail*. The newspapers named many of those mentioned in the report—the Royal Colleges, charities and the big regional councils—and share prices in tobacco companies fell slightly when trading on the Stock Exchange opened on Monday.

However, there was angry reaction from some of those advisers the BMA had been relying upon during its campaign. They complained they had not been warned their organizations would be named. Cary Spink of the British Heart Foundation was one of those who had been closely involved in the campaign. 'The Foundation was upset', she said. 'We were supposed to be kept informed. We did not know that Grand Met had a holding in an American tobacco company and I think the Foundation and other involved organizations should have been given the opportunity to dispose of shares in Grand Met immediately'.

Twenty-four hours later the backlash was well under way. Tuesday's edition of the *Daily Telegraph*[1] carried a lengthy article under the headline 'BMA attacked for tobacco share black-list of health bodies'. This was based largely on the reaction of the Royal College of Surgeons of England, which admitted that it held tobacco-linked investments but added, 'It is not a perfect world'. An unrepentant spokesman for the College was quoted as saying: 'We don't feel we are actively supporting the tobacco industry. If we did apply a selective investment policy then we would not be doing our best for the college's finances'. The spokesman added sharply that he hoped Dr Havard did not get his milk from Express Dairy or go to a Berni Inn for a steak or on a Warner holiday, because they were all companies that come under the Grand Metropolitan umbrella.

The National Council for Voluntary Organisations, which had 2000 shares in the Imperial Group and 18,500 in Grand Met, said it thought the organization might go against court rulings if it did not find the most profitable investment for its clients.

Glasgow District Council, which was involved in the Glasgow 2000 campaign to make the city non-smoking by the end of the century, said it would keep its £390,000 shareholding in the Imperial Group but seek to encourage the company to diversify its activities. With an Imperial Group factory in the city, the council was anxious not to create unemployment.

In an aggrieved letter to *The Times*,[2] David Innes Williams, chairman of the council of the Imperial Cancer Research Fund, described as 'deplorable' the BMA's suggestion that there was a lack of common purpose among the health institutes 'which does not in fact exist'. He criticized the policy being advocated by the BMA as 'purist' and went on: 'The simplistic BMA view of the complexity of financial interest and markets invites a rejoinder that this august body would be better advised to concentrate on medical rather than financial and moral issues. The matter will be discussed in our finance committee. But how much more dignified and less inflammatory it would have been had the BMA approached us direct rather than through the press'. When it met at the end of January, the Research Fund decided to keep its £500,000 worth of shares in Grand Metropolitan, at least until they could be sold profitably.

However, other bodies announced that they were selling their shares. The British Heart Foundation said it would sell all its 36,000 shares in Grand Metropolitan[3] and the Foundation's director general said it was completely unaware that Grand Met had any association with the tobacco industry. Mind, the National Association for Mental Health, and the Royal College of Nursing also said they would be selling all their tobacco shares, while other organizations, such as the

NSPCC (National Society for the Prevention of Cruelty to Children), the Medical Research Council and the Medical Protection Society, said they would be reviewing their holdings.

So the report achieved much of what it set out to do even though many feathers were ruffled in the process. Senior consultants' representatives at the BMA were furious that the Association had published the report, upsetting eminent medical schools, Royal Colleges and, more importantly for them, hospitals and health authorities for whom they worked. Although many saw the decision to publish as a mark of the new-style BMA, it was in fact in the best radical tradition of the old-style BMA of the 1930s and 1940s. However, it was recognized after the Red Book controversy that the Association was using up a lot of credibility it had achieved over the years with other health bodies and Royal Colleges.

One clear indication that the BMA's campaign was making an impact was the attention being devoted to it by newspaper leader writers, a breed of anonymous opinion formers whose influence on other people's opinions has always been a subject for much speculation. On this occasion their attention to the BMA was distinctly critical. The *Daily Express*,[4] for instance, under the headline 'Meddling doctors', criticized the Association for 'sounding off on all kinds of topics'—a somewhat ironic criticism for a leader writer!—and for 'simplistic moralizing', and it concluded with the words 'Save us from the Dr Scargills of this world'. Elsewhere the BMA was described as the Esther Rantzen of the medical world—'aggressive, pushy and holier than thou'.[5]

Critical comments such as these were inevitable in the light of the robust campaign being waged. Wherever possible, however, Association officials attempted to reply to the criticism through newspapers' letters columns. No attempt had yet been made to try and seek the active support of newspapers by talking directly to their editors, leader writers and health correspondents. This was to come later.

REFERENCES

1. *Daily Telegraph*, 15 January 1985.
2. *The Times*, 16 January, 1985.
3. *Financial Times*, 15 January, 1985.
4. *Daily Express*, 17 January, 1985.
5. *Medical News*, 24 January, 1985.

A YOUNG DOCTOR FIGHTS BACK

At the centre of the BMA's campaign were a group of people on whom Pamela Taylor relied for advice. The idea of having a circle of informal contacts was first used by the BMA in the mid-1970s during the battle against the Labour Government's attempt to abolish pay beds. It was used again in the campaigns on the Police and Criminal Evidence Bill and the Data Protection Bill in 1983 and on the issue of prescribing the contraceptive pill to under age girls. In all these cases it proved highly effective. With the tobacco campaign, the BMA found it extremely useful to try to coordinate what other bodies were doing. This often involved the BMA and these organizations being prepared to give up some of their own sovereignty, but no formal commitments were demanded from any organization.

The advisers were a loose alliance of organizations and individuals, some of whom were more active than others. From ASH were David Simpson and deputy Patti White. The charities were represented by Nigel Kemp of the Cancer Research Campaign, Cary Spink of the British Heart Foundation and Amanda Jordan of the Spastics Society. Alison Dunn was involved from the Royal College of Nursing and Professor Charles Fletcher from the College of Health. Others included Debbie Bartley, a community physician from the Lewisham and North Southwark health authority, Dr Donald Lane of the Oxfordshire health authority and the Royal College of Physicians, Dr Godfrey Fowler from the department of community medicine and general practice at Oxford University and member of the RCGP and Dr Bobbie Jacobson, from the London School of Hygiene and Tropical Medicine former deputy director of ASH and author of *The Lady Killers*, a book on women and smoking.

The wealth of knowledge and experience brought together by these individuals was considerable. Some, like Professor Fletcher, had been involved in the smoking issue for over 20 years and had become world renowned. He was secretary of the Royal College of Physicians committee which in 1962 produced the report *Smoking and Health*, now recognized as a landmark in the fight against smoking. He was delighted with his new involvement. 'I felt it was very good having the BMA planning to take a really active interest', he commented.

Dr Fowler was a GP and an epidemiologist who had researched the morbidity and mortality of smoking, but the two key advisers were David Simpson and Simon Chapman, a leading anti-smoking campaigner from Australia on secondment to the Health Education

Council. Together with Pamela Taylor and John Dawson they formed an inner quartet who tended to mastermind events.

Chapman's presence was entirely fortuitous, but proved to be crucial in bringing Australia's considerable experience in anti-smoking campaigns to strengthen the BMA. It was sheer coincidence that he happened to be on an 18-month secondment with the HEC at the time the BMA decided to embark on its own campaign. When Pamela Taylor was planning the campaign, she was lent a copy of an Australian anti smoking pamphlet, *The Lung Goodbye*, written by Chapman, a research fellow at the Australian national health and medical research council. When she discovered he was in London, she immediately contacted him and recruited him to the BMA's cause.

Chapman and the other advisers were used primarily to liaise on activities such as deputations to Government departments, television and radio interviews or writing to the press. 'We work out together who is going to do what and when', said Pamela Taylor. 'It's coordinating all anti-smoking activities'. In this way any unnecessary duplication of effort was minimized. Individuals and organizations were kept in touch with the BMA's activities and future plans and the BMA was told about the plans of other organizations. There was a constant cross-fertilization of ideas, although some of these never came to fruition—such as the idea of launching a campaign song at a No Smoking disco, or asking television viewers to 'Spot a Violation' during TV programmes and fill in coupons to be sent to the broadcasting authorities. Failure to follow these ideas through was usually because of logistical problems or lack of manpower, but this was more than outweighed by the scale of the things that were happening.

By now, more than 250 *BMA News Review* readers had asked to be put on the association's special register of doctors willing to help in the campaign. They were sent a questionnaire about conditions in their areas and details of action they could take. Involving these new volunteer campaigners became an important factor in the battle. The BMA had learnt from ASH that as soon as it had persuaded a doctor to write a letter it had successfully broken the first spasms of inactivity. As Pamela Taylor put it, 'Doctors are going to feel lonely out there'. So she began to send out regular newsletters with thoughts and ideas, plus progress reports.

Many doctors took their own individual action. Dr J. G. Avery, district medical officer with South Warwickshire Health Authority, wrote to his area's three local MPs enclosing statistics for the number of deaths locally attributable to smoking—more than 400 a year. 'Many of these smokers die 10 or 20 years before their time', he wrote. 'Their illnesses put considerable pressure on our much needed bed space and cause a considerable increase in costs to the health service'. In Gloucestershire the county council ordered a ban on all cigarette advertising on council-owned property after one of its members, Dr Clive Froggatt, a Cheltenham general practitioner, urged councillors to set the public an example. 'I think it is absolutely disgraceful', he said, 'that we should be profiting from a practice which is known to cause thousands of deaths a year'.

The BMA was receiving many inquiries from the public and calls of support. Students wrote in asking for help with projects and teachers sought advice about effective health campaigns. At least one poem had been contributed as well as a campaign song. The West Midlands Regional Health Authority invited Dr Havard to its executive box at West Bromwich Albion, the first division no smoking football team it sponsored.

From the publicity point of view, the biggest impact came from the black-edged cards. Thousands had now been distributed by the BMA to doctors all over the country and many were beginning to find their way back to MPs at the House of Commons. Manchester GP, Dr Hilary Harris, for instance, sent in five cards to her MP, Alf Morris, within the first month and received an acknowledgement for each of them.[1] The causes of the five deaths she recorded were carcinoma of the larynx, carcinoma of the lung with cerebral metastases, myocardial infarction, ischaemic heart disease and a cerebral vascular accident.

However, it was one particular card which attracted a sudden spate of controversy. Dr Michael Ingram, a young GP trainee working in the cardiac department at Battle Hospital in Reading, sent a card to his MP and found he received more than an acknowledgement. For Sir William van Straubenzee, Conservative MP for Wokingham, took exception. He publicly branded the card as 'monstrous and totally unacceptable', 'dramatic and extremely ghoulish'.[2]

In a letter to Dr Ingram, Sir William demanded to be given the name and address of his constituent who had died so that he could investigate the matter carefully. 'I appreciate, of course, that this request will cause distress to the relatives of the deceased', he wrote. 'I very much regret this. But it is you and not I that has chosen to give publicity to the death of my constituent'. The MP, who admitted to being a moderate smoker, told his local newspapers 'I shall hunt Dr Ingram, I will make life very troublesome for him even if I have to draw attention to him through Parliament'.

Sir William, a senior Conservative backbencher and former Minister who was known in the House of Commons as 'The Bishop' because of his interest in ecclesiastical issues, was also well known locally for his occasional bursts of public outrage. Less well known, however, was the fact which emerged during this publicity that he had once acted as the parliamentary adviser for a public relations firm whose clients included the Tobacco Advisory Council.

A weaker soul than Dr Ingram might have wilted under the ferocity of Sir William's onslaught, but the young doctor was to prove a worthy adversary. He refused to back down and wrote to the Wokingham MP 'I am sorry you have misinterpreted the postcard's intention to draw your attention to the number of your constituents dying because of tobacco-related disease'. He said that under no circumstances would he supply Sir William with the name and address of his constituent who had died and added that if Sir William was to visit Battle Hospital he would show him 'far more ghoulish sights' as a result of the tobacco industry. 'The ghoulishness of the card is nothing compared to the ghoulishness of a patient suffering because of tobacco'.

Sir William's protests led West Berkshire Health Authority to advise Dr Ingram to stop sending out the BMA's cards with the name of the hospital on them, but by now the MP's tactics were proving counter productive. Local doctors, angry at Sir William's bombastic approach, were going out of their way to send black-edged cards to him whenever possible. National publicity had been given to the BMA's campaign, the local publicity had boosted the cause of anti-smoking in the Reading area and the hounding of Dr Ingram had converted the young doctor into the most zealous anti-smoking campaigner. As events were to show, Dr Ingram was to emerge a few months later as the founder of a new organization, an anti-smoking group adopting direct action as one of its weapons.

The controversy over the black-edged cards illustrated once again the toughness of the BMA's campaign. The cards were not popular with all doctors, nor indeed with all those individuals and organizations involved in the campaign, but never before had the Association adopted such a consistently hard and uncompromising approach. One example of this was that it had deliberately gone out of its way to risk a defendable libel action from the tobacco industry. At their press conferences, BMA officials no longer couched their language in traditionally moderate terms. Instead of referring to illness, they spoke of death and laid the responsibility for this directly at the door of the tobacco companies. 'We were advised that this could be defamatory, but we believed it would be possible to defend it', said Pamela Taylor. However, not a flicker came from the tobacco companies, no doubt because the prospect of fighting a libel action in the courts based on the available medical evidence was not appealing. The BMA's aggression, however, did not appear to be having any outward effect on the Government. Two days after publication of the Red Book on investment in the tobacco industry, Kenneth Clarke, the Minister of State for Health, appeared on Channel Four's 'Face the Press' programme and said he did not believe in the effectiveness of an advertising ban.[3] He said that Ministers were accused of giving in to the tobacco lobby if they did not agree with well-intentioned theories that an advertising ban would lead to a great drop in smoking. 'Actually I disagree with the effectiveness of that', he said.

Where the BMA was quite clearly winning was in the whole area of publicity. In the three months since the campaign had started, the number of anti-smoking stories appearing in the press had increased and not all, by any means, had been prompted by the BMA. One story which received considerable publicity at this time was Princess Margaret's visit to hospital for a small operation on her lung and the advice she received from her doctors to give up smoking—advice that she was shortly to ignore in the full glare of more publicity.

REFERENCES

1. *Pulse*, 8 December 1984.
2. *Reading Standard*, *Wokingham Times*, 17 January 1985.
3. *The Times*, 16 January 1985.

LESSONS FOR CAMPAIGNERS

Go to outside organizations and experts for advice and guidance

Check with others outside your organization. There are many organizations and individuals with considerable campaigning experience and impressive track-records, so ask for their help. It is naive to assume that a campaign—even if it has started successfully—can do without the advice of others.

Try to get as wide a network of supporters as you can

Keep communicating with them, using newsletters and/or your house publication(s). Identify simple but effective activities for them to do. Build on their willingness to help and spend time devising ways in which they can demonstrate their support. In turn support them and be positive not defensive.

Encourage the public to take part

Provide interested members of the public with up-to-date information and suggest ways in which they may help. Carefully go through letters from the public supporting your activities in case there are any useful suggestions. With hostile letters, analyse the arguments against you, and develop counter arguments.

Turn opposition to your advantage

The black-edged cards provoked public anger from an MP, and we used this in the local media to draw attention to the campaign.

MEETING THE SPORTS MINISTER

The BMA believed that its best chance of securing Government action on smoking lay in the area of sports sponsorship. While a ban on all tobacco advertising was seen privately as a long-term hope, legislation to phase out and eventually ban the sponsorship of sport by tobacco companies and end the voluntary agreement on sponsorship were regarded as much more attainable.

A voluntary agreement between the Government and the tobacco industry on the sponsorship of sport first came into operation in December 1977. The agreement was for a period of 'at least three years', but in December 1980 the then Minister for Sport Hector

Monro announced that after consultation with the Secretary of State for Social Services he had agreed with the industry that the agreement should continue for another year. In March 1982 a revised voluntary agreement was announced by the new Minister for Sport Neil Macfarlane.[1] Its main features were that:

— it should run until at least 31 December 1985,
— the existing expenditure ceiling, namely the actual expenditure in 1976 adjusted for inflation, to be maintained,
— Government health warnings to appear on press and poster advertising for, and on agreed static promotional signs at, sponsored sporting activities,
— the Minister for Sport to be informed by the companies of their sponsorship plans and any changes in those plans,
— the companies to consult with the Minister for Sport on any proposal to sponsor a sport not previously sponsored by the industry,
— activities in which the majority of the participants are under 18 years of age not to be sponsored by the companies,
— the companies to continue to sponsor non-televised minor and amateur activities,
— the companies to use their best endeavours to keep expenditure on media advertising and promotional activities within a reasonable proportion of total sports sponsorship expenditure.

It was to urge the Sports Minister to end this agreement that a BMA-led delegation of senior doctors went to the Department of the Environment on 7 February 1985 to see Neil Macfarlane.

In the party were BMA president Sir Douglas Black, the chairman of Council Dr John Marks, the chairman of the Board of Science and Education Professor Peter Quilliam, BMA secretary Dr John Havard and Dr John Dawson. With them was the president of the Royal College of Physicians Sir Raymond Hoffenberg.

The meeting opened with Dr Marks referring to the medical profession's belief that smoking was responsible for many deaths and the fact that the Government had accepted the dangers to health of smoking when it instituted the health warnings on cigarettes. He said the profession was particularly concerned about the effect of indirect advertising of products through sports sponsored by tobacco companies. He gave as an example the Benson and Hedges snooker championship which had been televised the previous week and where the name of the product was seen clearly but the players' bodies had obscured the health warning below. Dr Marks referred to the research by Dr Frank Ledwith showing that this type of sponsorship had raised the level of awareness of cigarette brand names among children and teenagers who watched such events. Sir Raymond Hoffenberg mentioned the Royal College of Physicians' report, *Health or Smoking*, and the increase in lung diseases as a result of the smoking habit in the older generation. Although older people in general were giving up, this was mainly in classes 1 and 2. In classes 4 and 5 this was not so, and these were the people who were most likely to be watching snooker and darts on television. Although adults in general were smoking less as a result of health education, more children were smoking.

The Minister agreed that adults had heeded the warnings about smoking and, although it was difficult to judge the situation relating to young people without a detailed survey, he accepted the profession's view that there had been a marked increase in smoking by 9 to 11 year-olds. Dr Havard referred to the impact of legislation introduced in Norway to ban the advertising of all tobacco products which had shown that though the effect on smoking in all age groups was not very significant, it had proved very effective in reducing the incidence of smoking of 11 to 16 year olds. The BMA's policy was that legislation should be introduced in the United Kingdom to ban the advertising of tobacco products, and the Norwegian experience had shown that it was effective. Macfarlane replied that he could not anticipate what the Government or Parliament would do, but he would not seek to deny that there was some impact on young people from the increase in televised sporting events. One of the department's civil servants present added that if complaints were made about advertising at sponsored events they would be followed up. Macfarlane said that the subject of logos had been raised with manufacturers. These were a gross violation of the voluntary code. He said he would draw the attention of the Tobacco Advisory Council to the matter. When the voluntary agreement with the council had been negotiated it had been made clear that the Government health warning should be visible in order that the subliminal effect of the product name would be eliminated to some degree.

The Minister then introduced the subject of alcohol, and he was to refer to it again later in the meeting. He expressed his concern about its increasing availability at sporting events and the deterrent effect on parents taking their children to such events. Dr Havard replied that this was alcohol abuse, but that cigarette smoking was an abuse of health. He said there was considerable concern in the medical profession about alcohol abuse. The Royal College of Psychiatrists had produced one report and was preparing another and the Royal College of Physicians also had a working party on the subject.

Macfarlane then turned specifically to the issue of sponsorship and said that encouragement should be given to bodies other than tobacco companies, such as finance companies. He himself had tried to encourage and influence such matters, but the market had to decide. The State did not run sport. That was a matter for the governing bodies. Where violations occurred, these were taken up with the Tobacco Advisory Council and with the individual companies. However, there were particular difficulties when a sponsoring company handed the advertising to an agency. One breach had occurred because the agent had known nothing about the voluntary agreement.

The Minister said that about 20 sports were involved, very few of which were wholly sponsored by tobacco companies. He said he had received requests to amend the voluntary agreement and also to change the titles of sporting events, although this latter point was a matter for the governing bodies of the sports. He believed it was the role of the BMA and the Royal colleges to encourage these governing bodies to be more aware of their responsibilities.

He accepted the profession's view that it was important that children should not be encouraged to take up smoking and he appreciated the point made by Dr Havard about young people and the impact on them of advertising. However, he said it was difficult to see how anything could be done about participants in snooker championships smoking during matches.

The Minister concluded by assuring the delegation that there would be no widening of the terms of the voluntary agreement. There was a balanced way forward. He would not outlaw the sponsorship of sport by tobacco companies, but would remain very vigilant especially with the increase in televised sporting events in the summer. He emphasized that any formal complaints must be sent to him immediately, but he repeated that the Government had no plans for legislation.

Dr Havard, in his concluding remarks, said that in the event of legislation not being introduced during that session of Parliament the BMA would seek a further meeting with the Minister before any new voluntary agreement was made.

In a press statement issued by the BMA after the meeting Dr Havard commented: 'We reminded the Sports Minister that TV sponsorship of sporting events influences young people in deciding whether or not to start smoking. The code of practice which is up for renewal was clearly not having the desired effect to keep tobacco advertising off our television screens. It was necessary to legislate against all such forms of sponsorship of sport on our TV as has been done in some Scandinavian countries, where it has resulted in a significant reduction in the proportion of young people smoking cigarettes. The Minister could give no undertaking that the Government would be prepared to introduce or to support such legislation, but he did agree to give careful consideration to any further evidence we could produce, and he particularly asked for examples of abuse of the existing code of practice. He expressed great concern about recent abuses of the code.

'We explained to the Minister that the most important single issue we had for him was the need to discourage young people from starting to smoke. Large numbers of young people were being persuaded to take up the habit as a result of sports sponsorship on TV. The argument that sport will suffer from the removal of sponsorship by tobacco companies is untenable. The whole picture of sponsorship has changed in recent years and the money from tobacco companies accounts for less than 10 per cent of the total given to sports sponsorship. Athletics and swimming do not accept any money from the tobacco industry and both sports have no difficulty in finding other sponsors'.

The BMA had now met Ministers from both the Department of the Environment and the Department of Health and Social Security, the two Government departments directly responsible for the voluntary agreements with the tobacco industry. Neither meeting had produced any tangible sign of progress, but as Dr John Marks commented: 'It is like dripping away at a stone. It is a long drawn out process'. However, there was a third Government department more powerful than either the DHSS or the DoE whose interest in the smoking issue was purely financial. This was the Treasury. The enormous revenue derived by the Government from the tax on cigarettes, almost £5000 million a year, gave the Chancellor of the Exchequer a direct interest in the BMA's activities, but with the Budget just a month away it also gave the BMA an opportunity to write to the Chancellor. In a letter to Nigel Lawson, the BMA's secretary Dr Havard asked for 'a substantial increase' in the duty on cigarettes. 'It is now more than ever necessary', he wrote, 'to discourage children from taking up the habit, and we feel that a substantial increase in the duty in this year's Budget would act as an important deterrent'. Commenting on his letter, Dr Havard said:[2] 'Cigarettes are still cheaper in relative terms than they were in 1965. We are concerned particularly to deter children from smoking and we believe that an increase in price may prevent children from starting to smoke. Price is the single most important fact governing consumption of cigarettes and, in order to improve the health of the population of the country, we are asking for a large increase'.

As events were to show, the Chancellor did not satisfy the BMA in his Budget, but one Minister who did give a boost to the anti-smoking cause at the end of February was John Patten, the Parliamentary Under Secretary for Health. He announced[3] an extra grant of £500,000 for the Health Education Council to fund a special Spring campaign aimed at women smokers. Announcing this, Patten had this to say: 'During the 1950s, cigarette smoking among women rose substantially and stayed high until the 1970s. Although it has fallen from 37 per cent in 1978 to 33 per cent in the most recent survey, we are now seeing the effects of the earlier rise in increased smoking-related diseases among women. In addition to these diseases, which are common to both sexes, smoking among women poses some special problems. It can lead to complications in pregnancy and have adverse effects on the baby, and there is evidence that women using the contraceptive pill who also smoke increase significantly their risk of circulatory diseases'.

Patten added that with the extra grant the HEC would now be spending some £2½ million on anti-smoking programmes in 1984/5, but set against the £100 million being spent by the tobacco industry on promoting its products, this figure looked rather less impressive.

REFERENCES

1. Department of the Environment press notice, 3 March 1982.
2. BMA press statement, 13 February 1985.
3. DHSS press release, 26 February 1985.

LESSONS FOR CAMPAIGNERS

Take your case to the relevant Government Ministers

You can get a hearing if you show support for your case. Publicise carefully any visits to Ministers, and in particular your communications to them and their responses. Remember that a Minister's views may not be the same as his colleagues' or even with Governments. By seeing them you have a chance to persuade them to change their views, and to give them information they might otherwise not get.

Contact relevant civil servants

Civil servants are powerful. They remain as Ministers come and go and may have a long history of dealing with your subject. You may be helping civil servants brief their Ministers more thoroughly while tapping a good source of advice for your campaign.

Make contact with as many Government departments as possible

Many issues concern more than one department. For example, ask the Chancellor of the Exchequer to increase the duty on cigarettes or protest to the Minister of sports about sponsorship abuses.

THE AUSTRALIAN CONNECTION

When it came to the fight against the tobacco industry, anti-smoking campaigners in Britain had much to learn from Australia. There, the campaign against the industry had gone down a much more assertive and aggressive path. The fact that the BMA's campaign was able to learn from and build on this Australian experience was thanks to two men, Simon Chapman and Dr Arthur Chesterfield-Evans.

Simon Chapman was a research fellow at the Australian National Health and Medical Research Council, a consultant on the smoking control programme of the International Union Against Cancer in Geneva and a consultant to the International Organisation of Consumer's Unions at the Hague. He had come to Britain to complete his PhD on tobacco advertising. His value to the BMA during its campaign was that he was able to advise the Association about what courses of action might succeed based on his knowledge and experience of what had been tried elsewhere and failed. In March the BMA published a booklet written by Chapman intended as a briefing document for other campaigning organizations. Entitled *Cigarette Advertising and Smoking: A Review of the Evidence*, the document set out to expose the worthlessness of the case put up by the tobacco lobby.

It refuted the four main arguments used by the industry. The first was that it should be legal to advertise cigarettes if it was legal to sell them. This, said Chapman, was a convenient rule which used the issue of legality to obscure the issue of health and ignored the fact that if tobacco was invented tomorrow with all the information known about it available no Government would allow it to be sold. The industry's second claim was that tobacco advertising did not influence the total demand for tobacco but only redistributed the market share among competing brands. Chapman's response was that it was inconceivable that any industry would avoid trying to expand its market. By definition, advertising sought to maximize sales. The third claim was that tobacco advertising was aimed only at adult smokers and not at children. Yet Chapman pointed out that tobacco advertisements appeared in the media and were accessible to children. Children could see a billboard, read a newspaper or a magazine, watch television and listen to the radio in just the way that adult smokers did. Fourth was the industry's claim that cigarette advertising provided smokers with information which persuaded them to convert to 'safer' filtered and low-tar cigarettes. Advertising bans were therefore inimical to both freedom of information and public health. Chapman's reply to this argument was that few categories of advertising could provide consumers with so little information as cigarette advertising. 'What information is provided by the Marlboro man, by the slashed silk in the Silk Cut advertisements or by the cryptic Benson and Hedges series?' he asked.

His booklet went on to criticise the industry's own research on advertising and to look at the experience of the advertising ban in Norway. 'It is indisputable', he wrote, 'that the introduction of the ban in 1975 was associated with a further decline in smoking. Norwegian boys who had been smoking more before the ban, smoked fewer cigarettes after its introduction'. He concluded: 'The bottom line in all argument about alleged freedoms, the role of the state, and tobacco advertising is the appalling, unnecessary and totally avoidable health consequences of smoking. Those who believe that the epidemic of premature smokers' deaths matters less than the corporate health of the tobacco industry will doubtless be long remembered in the history of public health. Others have different priorities, and have equally direct arguments to oppose tobacco advertising. They need to say no more than the obvious truth that tobacco promotions seek to, and inevitably often succeed in, promoting smoking, which kills more than one million people world wide each year. If arguments remain to delay legislation banning tobacco advertising, they will have nothing to do with public health'. Although Chapman's booklet received little coverage in the press, its real importance was reflected elsewhere. It was sent to every MP at the House of Commons and became widely quoted by other campaigning organizations. In short, it became an invaluable source document.

The second Australian to help the BMA's campaign was Dr Arthur Chesterfield-Evans. He was regarded as one of Australia's leading campaigners and activists against the tobacco industry and one of a growing number of the Australian medical profession prepared to risk prosecution by 'refacing' tobacco advertisements with spray paint. He was an active member of the group known as BUGA-UP (Billboard Utilising Graffitists Against Unhealthy Promotions), which had operated in several states of Australia since 1979. Thousands of hoardings had been 'refaced' with messages against the tobacco industry. Turning 'Marlboro' signs into 'it's a bore' and 'Dunhill' to 'Lung Ill' proved to be a potent method of building public and political antipathy towards the tobacco industry in Australia. Since the group's formation, some 20 people had been arrested, including four doctors, a professor of education, artists and medical students, but all were acquitted or fined nominal sums. Dr Chesterfield-Evans was among those who had appeared in court, although the charges against him were eventually dropped. In March 1985 he arrived in Britain to address an international conference in Edinburgh on health education. Hearing that he was visiting the country, the BMA was quick to invite him to BMA House in London to discuss Australia's experience of direct action campaigning. It was, perhaps, no coincidence that three months later the first anti-smoking direct action groups in England were formed.

Meanwhile the BMA continued to pursue more traditional campaigning methods, and at a press conference on 8 March to launch Simon Chapman's report, the Association announced that its president elect, Lord Pitt of Hampstead, a London general practitioner, would be introducing a Private Member's Bill in the House of Lords to outlaw tobacco advertising. Lord Pitt was due to take over the presidency of the BMA from Sir Douglas Black in July. Born in the West Indies, he had been active in British politics for over 20 years as a Labour member of the old London County Council and then the Greater London Council, before becoming its chairman. Now as a life peer in the House of Lords, he was to become a valuable voice for the BMA. Like the Bill introduced in December by Roger Sims, Lord Pitt's legislation stood no chance of being implemented, but unlike the Sims Bill, it was to prove luckier in the queue for debate 10 weeks later.

March also saw the introduction of Chancellor Nigel Lawson's second Budget. In it he announced that the tax on cigarettes would go up by 6p, an increase that did not satisfy the BMA, although Labour MP Laurie Pavitt took the view that but for the BMA's pressure there would have been no increase at all. In a press statement on the day of the Budget, 19 March, a BMA spokesman commented: 'So far as adults are concerned, 6p a packet on cigarettes is still not enough to give people the incentive they need to stop smoking while still ensuring that the Government is able to collect the revenue it wishes from this tax. The Department of Health's own figures show that 20p on a packet would only reduce the consumption by 2 per cent. As far as children are concerned—and it has been estimated that British children between the ages of 11 and 16 spends £60 million a year on smoking—it will be a stronger disincentive as children have less money to spend'. The following day, the first day of Spring, had been designated National No Smoking Day by a dozen medical organizations, including the BMA. It was estimated that more than two-and-a-half million people again tried to give up smoking and more than a hundred events took place around the country to help them do so.[1]

Further support for the BMA came at this time from the results of a National Opinion Poll[2] on smoking showing that more 18 to 24 year olds were smoking in 1984 than in 1981—41 per cent compared with 37 per cent. However, only 35 per cent of those who smoked were smoking more than 16 cigarettes a day, which was slightly better than in 1981 when half smoked more than 16 a day. Among the population as a whole there was little change in the percentage of smokers, but there was a slight fall among those aged 25 to 49 (46 per cent to 43 per cent) and an increase among those aged 50 to 60 (40 per cent to 43 per cent). The average age for young people starting to smoke was 12. The poll showed that more GPs were advising their patients to stop smoking and that people were trying hard to give up. In 1984 one in four smokers claimed to have given up for over a week three times or more. Five per cent of former smokers gave up because their GP had told them to, 32 per cent for health reasons and 23 per cent to save money.

Renewed evidence in the poll that young people had been influenced to start smoking by tobacco sponsored sporting events provided further ammunition for the BMA in its attempt to persuade the

BBC and the Independent Broadcasting Authority to take action to stop current abuses. Of the two, the BBC was by far the more important target. In 1983 the Corporation's two television channels had carried 283 hours of tobacco sponsored sport compared with just 18 hours carried by independent television. So early in April the BMA went to Broadcasting House in London to put its case directly to the BBC. With Dr Havard and Dr Dawson went John Hitchins, head of public affairs at the HEC. From the BBC were Bill Cotton, managing director of BBC Television, Cliff Morgan, head of outside broadcasts, and David Holmes, secretary of the BBC.

However, despite a pleasant and convivial lunch, the BMA was not able to win any promises from the BBC. The Corporation's officials admitted that they would be very happy not to cover tobacco sponsored events, but they had to compete with independent television. If an agreement existed between the BBC and the IBA, the body responsible for independent television, the BBC would be happy to abide by it, but in their view this was a matter for the Government. At a time when the BBC was having considerable problems over its funding and was facing strong pressure from the Government on the issue of advertising, it was clear that sports sponsorship was not one of its major preoccupations. But the BMA had at least made its point. Dr John Dawson commented: 'We know there are people from the tobacco companies who actually attend these events and take the cameramen out and buy them drinks. Consequently they tend to get the camera shots and angles they want. We don't do that'. However, the BMA was hopeful that pressure centrally would begin to filter its way down to what happened on the ground.

The BBC meeting was followed up by a similar visit to the IBA by Pamela Taylor and John Hitchins in an effort to persuade the authority to consider a concordat with the BBC on sports sponsorship. Although the door was not closed completely on the idea, the BMA again came away empty handed.

REFERENCES

1. *Daily Telegraph*, 3 April 1985.
2. *BMJ*, 16 March 1985.

LESSONS FOR CAMPAIGNERS

Enlist public sympathy

Attach well-known figures to your campaign organization and to your events and publicity. Have a Royal patron if possible or an eminent person as chairman. Involve leading actors or sports stars in campaign events or stunts. You may also associate stars with your messages, as tobacco campaigners did with Humphrey Bogart's tough image and death from lung cancer.

Produce publications to support your campaign

You should acquire specialist knowledge on different aspects of the campaign to use it to produce publications which will help your supporters and win over your opponents. Make sure they are competently produced, with positive wording and wide distribution. Use professionals whenever you can. Try to arrange accompanying publicity. Your house journal will be a useful place to start.

Take your argument to those who aid your opponents

Organizations such as the BBC and IBA may claim they do not promote cigarettes, but you will know from watching television that cigarette brand names are a common feature. Don't be put off by the thought, 'They will never give in'. Prepare your facts and go and see them. And keep at them.

Learn from campaigners abroad

Successes and failures vary from country to country, so make contact with key people and learn from them. Successful ideas can be taken and tried, unsuccessful ones should be analysed and modified. Keep in touch.

Concentrate on the areas your organization is qualified to speak about

The BMA's expertise is in medicine. We therefore opposed the promotion of tobacco related products and the introduction of Skoal Bandits (snuff dipping), which provided an added opportunity to make political capital.

Keep MPs informed

A further early day motion gives an excuse for campaigners to approach their local MPs again. The more signatories the better, and there may now be more information to give to the MP. You can also use this opportunity to establish whether the MPs stance has changed.

THEATRICAL SUPPORT AND A ROYAL SMOKER

April saw the emergence of a new organization, the Artists' Campaign Against Tobacco Sponsorship (ACTS). It was launched at a BMA press conference at BMA House by Actor Warren Mitchell, better known to millions as television's Alf Garnett, along with fellow actor Robert Mill and Sir Roy Shaw, former secretary general of the Arts Council, who had written an article for that month's *BMA News Review*. The new body aimed to seek pledges from theatres and sports organizers saying that they would no longer accept cash from the tobacco industry. The group was supported by a host of stars, among them Derek Jacobi, Rachel Kempson, Spike Milligan, Miriam Margoyles and Paul Eddington, who had resigned the previous year from the Bristol Old Vic's board of governors in protest at a £20,000 tobacco sponsorship deal. All of them said they would refuse to act in any production sponsored by a tobacco company.

At the press conference Sir Roy Shaw replied to the frequently heard argument that the arts and sport would be severely harmed if tobacco sponsorship were banned. He said that between £8 million and £10 million a year was given to sport by tobacco companies and about £1.25 million to the arts, but this total was a tiny proportion of the £130 million spent in this area by the Government on subsidies and the £1.054 million spent by local authority on subsidies. Moreover, it was a sum which the government could and should easily make good from the £4.5 billion a year it took in tobacco taxes. Sir Roy, who was secretary general of the Arts Council from 1975 to 1983, argued strongly that sport and the arts could survive perfectly well without tobacco sponsorship. In his *BMA News Review* article he wrote: 'I sympathize with those who are driven by poverty to accept tobacco money, but it is surely wrong to use the life enhancing image of arts and sports to put a glamorous mask on the ugly face of a life diminishing product'. Speaking at the press conference he added: 'The idea that the arts will take money from just anyone is nonsense. It would not take money from the IRA or heroin pushers, but tobacco kills more people than the two together'.

A survey by Sports Sponsorship Computer Analysis Ltd, produced for the first time at the press conference, showed that although tobacco companies invested less in sports sponsorship than many other companies they managed to dominate much of the highly valued television coverage. Other companies would therefore be only too willing to step into the breach if tobacco sponsorship were banned.

At the same time tobacco sponsorship of the arts came under attack from a group of MPs in the House of Commons. An early day motion drawn up by the BMA and sponsored by MPs from all parties urged the Government 'to take action to curb the promotional activities of a product from which 100,000 die prematurely each year, by banning all forms of sponsorship of the arts by tobacco companies, and in view of the fact that tobacco sponsorship of the arts forms only 10 per cent of the total sponsorship and its loss would not harm the funding of the arts, to encourage arts organizations to accept sponsorship from alternative sources'. The motion was sponsored by Conservative MPs Roger Sims (Chislehurst) and Nigel Forman (Carshalton and Wallington), Labour MPs Jack Ashley (Stoke on Trent South) and Alf Dubs (Battersea), John Cartwright (Woolwich) from the Social Democrats and Clement Freud (Cambridgeshire North East) for the Liberals.

Alf Dubs, commenting on the motion,[1] said: 'I have enormous sympathy for the arts and I will work to get money from virtually any source to help them. But sponsorship of the arts by tobacco companies is against the spirit of the agreement between the Government and the tobacco industry and it associates the arts with something which kills so many people each year. It is totally unacceptable and the arts will have to find money from elsewhere for its support'.

The lure of tobacco cash, however, remained strong. A spokesman for the Arts Council was reported as saying: 'Smoking is not against the law and therefore we are happy to accept tobacco sponsorship and would be very unhappy to lose it. The arts need every penny they can get'.[2]

From Scotland came news of a similar inducement in the sporting field. At the end of the Air Canada Silver Broom curling world championship in Glasgow, organizers of the sport in Scotland spoke confidently about the rapid growth of curling in the country thanks to new ice rinks being built with curling facilities. One was planned for Aberdeen with the help of £14,000 to be put up by the tobacco company Benson and Hedges. Mrs Alison Hillhouse, Scottish director of ASH, described the company's move as 'cynical and shocking, but not surprising', while a BMA spokesman said it was 'another attempt to buy phoney respectability for their killer products'.[3]

However, undoubtedly the most beneficial publicity derived by the anti-smoking campaign at this time came from the direction of the Royal Family. On the very day of the BMA's press conference launching ACTS, Princess Margaret was photographed across London smoking at a reception at Grosvenor House.[4] Just three months after her stay at the Brompton Hospital where a small piece of her left lung had been removed, the 54-year-old Princess was seen smoking her favourite untipped cigarettes in her familiar tortoiseshell holder, despite medical warnings from her doctors to abandon the habit. The following morning's newspapers gave the event full coverage.

Ironically, Labour MPs were still campaigning hard for an end to the Royal Warrant being granted for certain cigarette brands. Ernie Roberts, chairman of the Labour Party's Parliamentary Health Committee, had called earlier in the year for a withdrawal of the warrant and had been strongly supported by the BMA. A Buckingham Palace spokesman said that all companies which had a Royal Warrant were vetted once a year in December and their warrants were continually under review.[5] This led a group of Labour MPs to table an early day motion in the Commons welcoming the news 'that her Majesty is reconsidering the Royal Warrant at present given to cigarette manufacturers and is delighted to learn that so many of the Royal Family are not in danger of contracting the chest and heart diseases which arise from the smoking habit'.

The unexpected benefit of publicity from the subject of Princess Margaret was more than offset for the BMA by a major new development which was to add a totally new issue to the campaign, as well as a new name—Skoal Bandits. Once again the junior members' forum was the first to voice the profession's concern. Meeting in Belfast at the end of March they demanded the banning of 'tobacco teabags'. Just two weeks later, on 18 April, the Department of Health announced that the Government had made an agreement with an American tobacco company to restrict the marketing of Skoal Bandits, described as 'an increasingly popular tobacco product which is sucked in a sachet in the mouth'.[6] The miniature sachet contained a small quantity of fine-cut moist tobacco and was held between the cheek and gum. It was sold widely in America and was already on sale in parts of the Midlands and the north of England. The DHSS said that the agreement with US Tobacco International ensured that marketing of Skoal Bandits was not directed at young people under 18 and non-smokers. The department had been advised that tobacco sucking, or snuff dipping as it was also known, increased the risk of cancer of the mouth.

In addition, the company had been asked to observe certain conditions in marketing Skoal Bandits or any similar products in Britain. These were embodied in a voluntary agreement reached between UK Health Ministers and the American company which would run until at least December 1987. Under its terms the marketing of the product would be specifically directed at adult tobacco users and restrictions were placed, among other matters, on advertising content and media, on free sampling and on the choice of retail outlets.

To accompany this announcement from the DHSS, Dr Donald Acheson, chief medical officer at the department, wrote to all doctors about the dangers associated with snuff dipping. He saw that medical evidence on the product had been studied by the department's committee on carcinogenicity and he went on: 'The committee found that the habit significantly increased the risk of developing cancer of the mouth, an extremely unpleasant disease which might be difficult to treat and could result in disfigurement or death'. Dr Acheson said that some smokers might be tempted to try snuff dipping either as a way of hoping to give up cigarettes or as an alternative to smoking, but he said they should be aware that while this habit was much less dangerous than cigarette smoking it could not be considered safe. His advice to smokers was that they should consider other safer methods of giving up smoking.

The BMA was astonished at the Government's announcement and reacted immediately by strongly criticizing the Department of Health for allowing the 'tobacco teabags' to go ahead. It described the agreement between the department and the company as farcical and completely inadequate and said it was 'a disgrace' that the Government had not banned the new product. As Pamela Taylor wrote in her campaign briefing letter to doctors: 'The irony of (Dr Acheson) writing to doctors while leaving children unprotected from the industry's promotional activities is evidently lost on the DHSS. Nobody is going to write to the children to tell them to close their eyes each time they see advertisements for this product'.

The controversy over Skoal Bandits was to become an important new strand in the BMA's campaign. The new product was to lead the campaign into the complexities of the legislation governing nicotine and poisons and the opening by the company of a Scottish factory in East Kilbride was to incense local doctors. Thus, what could have been a setback for the anti-smoking campaign became a bonus for the BMA.

REFERENCES

1. *Yorkshire Post*, 3 April 1985.
2. *Medical News*, 11 April 1985.
3. *Glasgow Herald*, 2 April 1985.
4. *Daily Telegraph*, 3 April 1985.
5. *Daily Express*, 25 April 1985.
6. DHSS press release, 18 April 1985.

WESTMINSTER ACTIVITY

The BMA's reputation as one of the country's most powerful lobbying organizations goes back many years. Earlier this century the social reformers Sidney and Beatrice Webb described the BMA as 'one of the most highly developed and most efficient of all British professional organizations'. However in recent years the BMA's lobbying activities had increased out of all recognition to the days of the Webbs, and one of the reasons for this growth and for the Association's greater political professionalism was the establishment of its parliamentary unit. Few organizations and pressure groups have the resources to set up a separate section dealing solely with parliamentary affairs, but in 1980 the BMA set out along this path by appointing Sue Marks as its first parliamentary officer. Her job was to monitor what was happening in Parliament so that BMA officials could be kept in touch with activities at Westminster and MPs and peers could be kept in touch with the views of the BMA. These contacts, built up over the next few years, were to prove crucial in the anti-smoking campaign. The constant monitoring of activity both in the Commons and the Lords enabled the BMA to identify potential allies as well as potential opponents, and to tailor its lobbying accordingly. Before it had a parliamentary unit, the Association used to mail all 635 MPs when it was concerned about an issue. Now with its more finely tuned knowledge of MPs' activities, it tended to contact only those Members interested in the subject.

Throughout the campaign the BMA kept in close touch with those interested MPs and peers of all parties. They were written to on a regular basis and sent copies of BMA News Review and the various campaign reports which had been published, and some MPs and peers were seen personally to be briefed. Only twice were all MPs contacted, once when they were sent Simon Chapman's booklet, to enable them to answer questions from their constituents, and again to seek support for an early day motion. Monitoring support for the various motions which were by now on the Commons order paper was another task for Sue Marks. The motion tabled by Roger Sims in November, 'Smoking and Children', had attracted the support of 58 other MPs in the two weeks after it had been tabled, but in February Dr Havard decided to write to all MPs asking for their support, and as a result the number of signatories rose to over 90. In April Roger Sims tabled his motion 'Tobacco Sponsorship and the Arts', primarily to coincide with the BMA's press conference that month. On this occasion only selected MPs were written to and the number of signatories remained at around the 30 mark.

BMA lobbying also led to a number of questions being tabled in both Houses.[1] The Liberal MP Michael Meadowcroft took up the case of Dr Ingram and the black-edged cards, Roger Sims asked about the voluntary agreements between the tobacco industry and the Government, and the veteran Labour MP Laurie Pavitt questioned Ministers on issues ranging from cigarette sales to the television coverage of sponsored sporting events—although not all his questions were as a result of prodding from the BMA.

In May the two BMA Bills were due to be debated—Roger Sim's Bill in the Commons to phase out tobacco sponsorship and Lord Pitt's Bill in the Lords to ban tobacco advertising. The BMA's strategy was to mount a two-pronged attack, each Bill seeking to achieve different ends, but the tactics employed on each were different. The Sims Bill, down for its second reading debate on May 10, was deliberately not preceded by any publicity or any extensive lobbying because there was virtually no chance of it being debated. It was purely a propaganda exercise. In the event it was not debated, though not because of any devious tactics by the tobacco lobby, but because all the available time was taken up on the previous Bill to outlaw kerb crawling.

Lord Pitt's Bill, however, was to fare rather better. It, at least, was debated, and on this occasion the BMA did what it could to mobilize support. The aim of the four-clause Bill was to phase out all tobacco advertising within a three-year period, a more limited goal than the BMA had originally intended, but the debate on May 22 was not a great success for the BMA. Not only did it lose the vote, it also lost much of the argument, largely because many of those peers who said they would speak for the Bill did not turn up. This probably had something to do with the fact that the debate was after 7 p.m., which in their lordship's view was unsociably late.

The debate lasted for almost two-and-a-half hours and was opened by Lord Pitt, who referred to the estimate that tobacco accounted for between 15 and 20 per cent of all British deaths. Yet apart from legislation to ban the sale of tobacco goods to children under 16 and the ban on cigarette advertising on television, the Government had so far refused to legislate on the subject. He reminded peers that he had first spoken on the subject of smoking and health in his maiden speech in 1975. In the 10 years since then, about one million people had died prematurely in the United Kingdom from the effects of smoking.

Lord Pitt's speech was followed by a succession of peers, many of whom confessed that they were smokers, who were strongly opposed to any legislation to ban advertising. The Conservative peer Lord Mottistone said there was no evidence that advertising caused anyone, including children, to start smoking, and Lord Kaberry of Adel, a former Conservative MP in Leeds, said the Bill was not to ban tobacco products but to ban the advertising of them and as such was a nonsense. The economist Lord Harris of High Cross described the Bill as 'at once trivial and yet heinous, breaching the sacred liberal principle that kept compulsion for use against major threats to the peace and security of a free society'.

The strongest support for the Bill came from Lord Pitt's fellow general practitioner Lord Rea, who practised from a health centre in London's Kentish Town. He said that for the Government to continue to allow advertising was in effect condoning the habit and legitimizing its continuation. The Countess of Mar said that although she smoked 20 to 30 cigarettes a day she supported the Bill. It might be too late for her, but if the House could stop others from taking their first cigarette, particularly children, it would have done a tremendous service. For the Government, the Earl of Caithness argued the case for health education rather than legislation. He claimed that the present code governing the advertising of cigarettes was working well. Lord Pitt's Bill, however, would create something of a precedent in introducing wide ranging statutory controls on the promotion of products which were themselves freely and legally available for sale.

At the end of the debate, Lord Pitt described himself as 'bloody but unbowed', but said that the most important point was the need to create an atmosphere in which non-smoking was regarded as the acceptable and preferable thing and smoking was not the desirable, respectable or preferable thing. However, on a vote, the House decided against giving the Bill a second reading by 26 votes to 11.

In the week after the debate, another parliamentary opportunity arose for the BMA to get its message across. The House of Lords, European Communities Committee was taking evidence on Britain's response to a European Commission document on the scope for social action and cooperation on health matters within the European Community. This document had suggested that there was scope for action on tobacco use, illicit drugs and infectious diseases. This gave the BMA the chance to submit evidence on smoking—and to gain further media publicity. The Association argued in its submission that tobacco and alcohol were killing more people than drugs. 'We accept that drug abuse is a problem which is given a huge amount of media attention. Nevertheless, at the moment the numbers of people involved are a fraction of those affected by the two other major addictions—smoking and alcohol abuse'.

Its evidence on tobacco read: 'Any initiative by the Commission in relation to smoking should be seen in the context of the history of the campaign in the United Kingdom. The British Medical Association's policy in relation to smoking dates from 1971. Since that date the Association, in conjunction with the other medical organizations and in particular the Royal College of Physicians, has been campaigning actively to increase the public awareness of the dangers of smoking.

'Although successes have been achieved, we believe that much more is needed. The present cigarette warnings are not effective. In many cases they are the only means by which a cigarette advertisement can be identified as such. We believe the warnings should come from the manufacturers themselves and should state the types of disease caused by cigarette smoking. The framework of the Treaty of Rome presents an ideal way to achieve the adoption of a code of advertising in relation to cigarettes which would assist in realizing a common approach by individual member states. It would also avoid problems such as different criteria for advertising on television which distorts advertising in the Community by trans-border influence.

'The voluntary code on advertising practice is ineffective and this association has launched a major campaign to put pressure on the industry and on the relevant authorities to stop advertising and the promotion of tobacco products. Both the BMA and the Health Education Council are maintaining a high level campaign to inform the public about the activities of the tobacco industry.

'There is now a developing problem in relation to the number of women smokers. The burgeoning female death toll from smoking-induced disease—which killed nearly 33,000 British women in 1983 from coronary heart disease, lung cancer and chronic bronchitis—reflects the large-scale growth of smoking among women since the last World War. While lung cancer is declining among men, it is rising inexorably among women and has already overtaken breast cancer as the biggest cause of death from cancer in women aged between 65 and 74. Smoking also imposes unique, increased risks for young women. Those who take the contraceptive pill and smoke have an increased risk of coronary heart disease and stroke (mainly subarachnoid haemorrhage). New evidence has also linked smoking to cancer of the cervix. Smoking is also known to harm the unborn baby and is linked to an earlier menopause. A Community initiative to tackle this problem is urgently needed.

'The Standing Committee of Doctors of the EEC has already stated in its declaration on preventive medicine that the doctors of the 10 member countries are ready to increase their contribution to appropriate programmes of measures to extend preventive medicine to the promotion of health and education for health.

'The BMA believes that the most urgent problems to be tackled are tobacco advertising, particularly advertising in women's magazines, and the sponsorship by the tobacco industry of sporting events. It must be recognized that different approaches may need to be used in the differing member states of the community due to the different social and cultural attitudes. Nevertheless, in the matter of education, the UK has most to offer the other member states and has already shown a good lead. The benefit of achieving a reduction in smoking amongst the population is measured not only in terms of reduced mortality but also in terms of a huge reduction in morbidity'.

The BMA's evidence concluded by saying that substances causing health problems such as tobacco, alcohol and drugs should be treated in the same way as a communicable disease. Tobacco was a good example in that the multinational manufacturers crossed borders and promoted products causing major mortality and morbidity. An effective coordinating organization was needed to counteract this influence.

Commenting on the BMA's evidence, Dr John Dawson said: 'The sickness caused by cigarette smoking is now so well known that the European Commission could take a major public initiative by requiring tobacco companies to accept liability for the disability and disease caused by their products'.[1]

REFERENCES

1. *Hansard*, 1 February, 29 March, 16 and 17 April 1985.
2. BMA press statement, 24 May 1985.

LESSONS FOR CAMPAIGNERS

Keep those speaking on your behalf fully briefed

Maintain contact with those MPs and Lords who pledge their support for your campaign and keep updating your information on those parliamentarians whose views are unknown. See them in person and write to them. If a parliamentary debate looks likely, ensure that whoever is promoting the Bill has all the information he/she needs—offer information to other supporters, encouraging them to take part in the debate.

Use every opportunity to attract publicity

Select Committees in the Commons and Lords monitor the work of Government departments. They often provide an opportunity for publicity when an organization is giving evidence. Parliamentary questions (PQs) can be tabled on many issues apart from the obvious; if you have a specific local difficulty a PQ can bring it out into the open.

A VOTE OF CONFIDENCE

In May 1985 the BMA, in conjunction with the Health Education Council, published its next report, *When Smoke Gets in Your Eyes*, on cigarette advertising in women's magazines. Written and researched by Dr Bobbie Jacobson, research fellow in health promotion at the London School of Hygiene and Tropical Medicine, and Dr Amanda Amos, senior scientific officer at the departments of community medicine and health education at Hampstead Health Authority in north London, the report revealed how the tobacco industry was breaching its voluntary agreement with the Government by aiming its promotions directly at girls and young women through women's magazines. At least one million non-smokers in the 15 to 24 age group were being exposed to advertisements for cigarettes in these magazines in violation of Government policy and nearly 60 per cent of magazines with a youthful readership profile accept cigarette advertisements. This was at a time when smoking among girls and young women was rising as well as the female death toll from smoking-induced diseases, which totalled almost 33,000 in 1983 and was still rising.

The report found that nearly two-thirds of the 53 women's magazines surveyed accepted cigarette advertising and few published articles warning of the dangers of smoking. Only 37 per cent of British magazines had recently given wide coverage to the topic or were planning to do so. In a preface to the report, Dr John Havard said there was evidence that editoial coverage of the dangers of smoking was likely to be compromised when magazines accepted cigarette advertising. The report called for legislation to ban all tobacco advertising and promotion, and in the meantime for the Advertising Standards Authority's code of practice to be strengthened so that cigarettes could no longer be advertised in any magazine whose largest readership group was under 25. The tobacco industry should be instructed to stop advertising immediately in youth magazines. The report also suggested action which could be taken by individuals ranging from contacting their local radio stations to give interviews on the subject, contacting MPs and writing to the Advertising Standards Authority and to editors of women's magazines.

The report received widespread press and television coverage, and upset the tobacco industry and the Advertising Standards Authority sufficiently to provoke some angry correspondence in the *New Statesman*, as well as a strong protest from Peter Thompson, the ASA's director general. The complete acceptance of the report's findings among magazine proprietors and editors was impressive by comparison. Indeed, *Good Housekeeping* praised the report in an editorial, and wished the BMA success in its efforts to get a ban on tobacco promotion. More significantly still, the report provoked a major review of cigarette advertising policy in all women's magazines owned by IPC—the biggest women's publishing group. This resulted in a decision being made at board level that no IPC magazine with a target readership age of 20 or less should accept cigarette advertising. This was a substantial victory as it led to *Honey* magazine, against the inclination of its editor, to terminate its contract with its cigarette advertisers.

Finally the document earned a footnote in BMA history as the first BMA report ever to be published simultaneously in electronic as well as printed form. Doctors with suitable computers could dial Data-Star's information service and read or print out the report. Personal computers could also be used by interested patients with the addition of low cost accessories.

As the campaign entered its ninth month, Pamela Taylor and senior BMA officials had every reason to feel pleased with the way things had gone. The whole campaign had been conducted entirely within BMA policy. Elected officers and BMA divisions had been kept informed of every stage by a steady stream of briefings from the Professional Relations Unit—and many had offered active support. However, now they had to face the test of the BMA's annual representative meeting where they knew that critics of the campaign would rightly have their say. The Association's annual meeting was in effect the doctors' Parliament, the Association's representative body where more than 600 doctors from all the specialities gathered to decide policy on the major medico-political and ethical issues of the day. This was the BMA's democratically elected policy making body and the venue for the 1985 conference was the Theatre Royal in Plymouth. The subject of smoking was due to be debated on the third day, 26 June. Among the 25 motions on smoking, only one was critical of the campaign.

A clear indication that the tobacco industry was now seriously worried about the impact of the campaign came on the eve of the conference when the Tobacco Advisory Council wrote to national newspapers expressing its willingness to comment on the issue. The letter noted the marked increase in the scale of the attack on cigarette advertising mounted by the BMA, ASH and other pressure groups and went on: 'There will be another round of criticism arising from the annual representative meeting of the BMA. The tobacco industry holds that its critics have a perfect right to advance their point of view, but we believe we also have every right to express our thinking on issues as important to us as product advertising and sponsorship. Perhaps we have adopted too low a profile in the past and our case may well have suffered by default. Some of the observations and opinions being expressed by those opposed to tobacco advertising are completely misleading and based upon emotive and quite irresponsible considerations. If the TAC, as the trade association representing the UK tobacco manufacturers, can help you with a comment on such matters, we shall be glad to give it—and fast'.

Clearly the tobacco industry had decided that the BMA was winning the argument, a view strengthened when the Tobacco Advisory Council's public affairs manager, Tony St Aubyn, told BMA News, 'The amount of anti-tobacco news floating about at the moment has persuaded my lords and masters that keeping your head down below the parapet is no longer a going concern. They want us to be more obvious and make ourselves more available'.

The BMA could have asked for no clearer evidence that its campaign was working and this was the message taken up by speaker after speaker when the debate on smoking took place at the Plymouth annual meeting. There was a certain justice in the fact that the debate was opened with a motion welcoming the campaign and urging that it should continue until its aims had been achieved, proposed by Dr Gabriel Scally, the young community doctor from Belfast who played such a significant part at the previous year's meeting. He had no doubt about the success of the campaign, but a small minority did. Dr Roy Hooper, a consultant from the Midlands, said he approved of most of the campaign but not the black-edged cards. 'Am I the only professional person who views this card device as utterly distasteful?' he asked. To judge by the silence from the hall he was indeed one of the very few. Another consultant, John Storrs from East Kent, said he had been keeping a rough check on the number of people at the conference lighting up, 'occasionally with stealth', outside the hall. His total so far was 58. 'I would suggest that some caution be exercised in how far the BMA goes down the road of wishing to deprive the individual adult of his option to smoke'. But Dr John Marks, replying on behalf of the BMA Council, said, 'The reason they do it with stealth is because they are actually ashamed of what they are doing at a BMA meeting'. As for the campaign, he said, 'I think we are doing it well. That is why there is so much screaming. We are winning slowly against a massive body with enormous funds'. Representatives at the conference clearly agreed with Dr Marks because on a vote they supported the campaign with only three against.

The conference then went on to debate motions calling for a Tobacco Act to ban all tobacco advertising and tobacco sponsorship of the arts and sport and increased penalties for shopkeepers selling cigarettes to children. Each motion was passed by a massive majority, only a handful of representatives voting against. Two of the BMA's stalwart members, consultant Dick Greenwood and ophthalmologist Michael Gilkes, raised their voices against the BMA's campaigning crusades to ban this and ban that and said it was not the Association they had joined—to which Dr Marks retorted 'I am glad to say it is not the Association I joined either. The Association I joined did nothing, acted on nothing and produced precious little'.

The issue of Skoal Bandits was raised by several speakers who produced the teabag and waved it in front of the conference for those doctors who had not seen one before. There was widespread agreement that the product should be banned as quickly as possible before it could gain a hold in Britain, but on another motion to ban smoking in public property used for NHS health care, representatives were divided, with several speakers pointing out that this would be cruel to a substantial minority of patients in psychiatric hospitals. The motion was eventually lost by 107 votes to 87.

At the end of the day Dr Havard told a press briefing that the debates were 'a complete vindication of the policies we have used to bring our views on smoking before the public'. He repeated that the voluntary agreements were not working and that a total ban on tobacco advertising and sponsorship was the only way.

However, as a public relations exercise, the conference was not entirely successful. The reason was that it also decided to call for a complete ban on alcohol promotion and advertising. This led to a flurry of press criticism about the BMA's 'ban everything' approach. Publicly, Dr Havard was not at all apologetic. 'The more we identify public health hazards and move in this direction, the more we are recognized as being aunties and trying to ban everything. Our track record shows that we do not call for things to be banned unless there is a very good public health reason, and when the necessary measures have been introduced and have been banned there is always a substantial spin off'. Privately, however, the Association's leaders accepted that to launch a major campaign on alcohol at the same time as they were campaigning heavily on smoking was neither wise nor practical.

The Plymouth conference was marked by one other announcement, which although not strictly part of the BMA's anti-smoking campaign, added greatly to the general anti-smoking aura which was now developing. After the previous year's annual conference debate when representatives voted to sever all BMA links with unit trusts investing in tobacco companies, senior officials of the Association had been working hard to find a way of putting this into practice. As a result, Tony Grabham, former chairman of the BMA Council and now chairman of BMA Services Ltd, was able to announce a new unit trust which guaranteed not to invest in the leading tobacco companies.

The service was to be launched jointly by BMA Services and Fidelity International Management and was to be called the Professional Growth Trust. A specific list of 'blacklisted' tobacco companies had been drawn up, six in the United Kingdom—BAT Industries, Rothmans International, Grand Metropolitan, Imperial Group, Molins and Bunzl—and 12 outside the UK—in America, American Brands, Culbro, Dibrell Brothers, Philip Morris, Loews Corporation, R. J. Reynolds, US Tobacco and Universal Leaf Tobacco, and in Europe, A. L. Van Beek, Rohte and Jiskoot, Obel and Amer. Special terms were to be offered to BMA members, although it was hoped that the trust would have a wider appeal than just to doctors.

Dr Gabriel Scally, the young doctor whose persistence had much to do with the setting up of the new trust, commented: 'I am of course absolutely delighted, if a little bemused, at the speed with which this has been done, given the amount of opposition to the subject last year'.

LESSONS FOR CAMPAIGNERS

Join with other organizations to promote publications

Link with others publicly. Often the differing expertise in two organizations can be brought together to produce a publication, and joint publications can have added impact. They can be accompanied by joint press conferences and joint activities in both Houses of Parliament.

Accept your responsibilities to your members and learn from their criticisms

Your authority to campaign comes from your members. Accept criticism. You are responsible to a formally elected body, listen to and learn from any criticisms.

Keep the press informed on internal discussion

Some formal meetings can be opened to the press. This is a useful way to get publicity, but you should be confident that the meeting will reach a decision worth publicising. Remember that participants react differently when the press are present, and that all the journalists may choose to publicise aspects of the debate you would rather keep quiet on. The alternative is to issue a statement, or hold a press briefing after a closed debate.

Don't be afraid to go public

Some negotiations (e.g. on the tobacco voluntary agreement) are in secret. This does not mean that organizations who submit evidence cannot publicise it.

Keep anticipating the opposition's moves

Never assume they are content with using existing channels. Look ahead and try to anticipate new approaches (e.g. new ways of promoting tobacco products) and then try to ensure you act first.

Take time out during the campaign to assess progress and plan fresh initiatives

How is all going? Build into your campaign planning sessions when short-, medium- and long-term goals can be reassessed. Small informal brain-storming sessions can be built on by inviting one or two outside experts to join. MPs and Lords are often willing to take part in planning sessions.

Watch out for political changes

Ministerial reshuffles can mean that views will change. Check the previous voting patterns of new Ministers, gauge their views and send a deputation to brief them. They may have different arguments from their predecessors, and different soft spots on which to play.

PHASE ONE ENDS, ANOTHER BEGINS

The Plymouth conference effectively marked the end of Phase One of the BMA's campaign. This coincided with the departure of one of the campaign's key organizers, Simon Chapman, whose secondment to the Health Education Council came to an end in June. Before leaving Britain to return to Australia, Chapman went to a small farewell party held for him by the BMA and attended by those who had campaigned so hard over the past eight months. There was a justifiable feeling of satisfaction at that gathering about what had been achieved since the start of the campaign the previous October. 'We knew that what we had done was to raise public awareness of the deaths and the scale of the problem we are talking about', said Dr John Dawson. 'What we were doing had made it more acceptable for doctors to do things and by publicising things we had tried to stimulate people'. Parliamentary activity had also been increased, and as a result the tobacco industry was now clearly worried.

An indication of this was the decision by the firm Alfred Dunhill to launch an international advertising campaign stressing that it had nothing to do with cigarettes.[1] The company found itself suffering from a public image which incorrectly perceived it to be a tobacco company. In fact the firm was founded in 1907 selling pipes and other smokers' requisites, including pipe tobacco, and it was Carreras Rothmans, as it was then known, which first started making Dunhill cigarettes under licence in 1952. Rothmans UK now had a 51 per cent shareholding in Alfred Dunhill, who received a royalty from the sale of Dunhill cigarettes, but whose main business was fashion and accessories.

Further evidence of the industry's growing concern came in July when the Tobacco Advisory Council produced a half-hour video and circulated a glossy brochure to Ministers and selected MPs putting its side of the case in preparation for the negotiations on the voluntary agreements. The brochure which proclaimed 1985 to be 'the year of decision', referred specifically to the BMA's campaign, prompting ASH's David Simpson to declare, 'This is the most tangible and transparent piece of evidence that the industry is on the run. If they were not worried they would not do anything'. At the same time it had to be admitted that ministerial opinion appeared firm. Action continued to be taken on the periphery, such as the Department of Health's circular in June instructing all health authorities to curtail smoking in hospitals and on all NHS premises.[2] However, with the coming negotiations in mind, Health Ministers were letting it be known that the idea of a total ban on tobacco advertising was a political non-starter. The repercussions would be too great. Their advice to the BMA was to concentrate on the sports sponsorship issue.

In a letter sent out by Pamela Taylor at the end of May to the 300 doctors who had registered as volunteers for the campaign, she had this to say: 'Although our ultimate aim is the introduction of a Tobacco Act prohibiting all promotional activity, this is not feasible yet. Our short term aim, therefore, is to stimulate debate on specific aspects of our campaign, forcing Parliament and press to take notice of doctors' views'.

Throughout the summer and autumn of 1985 the BMA, the Health Education Council, ASH and the Royal College of Physicians began to increase their activity as Ministers met the tobacco industry for the first of their preliminary meetings on new voluntary agreements. The BMA and the Royal College of Physicians asked for observer status at the negotiations. Dr Amanda Amos from Hampstead Health Authority followed by ASH exposed a new breach of the advertising rules, a four-page 'advertorial'—a photographic advertising feature—in the August edition of *Options* magazine.[3] The promotion was ostensibly for the liqueur Tia Maria and featured a young couple going out to dinner, but in each of the settings, the Raffles cigarette brand also appeared, posing as the name of a restaurant and as the cover of an LP record. Yet nowhere was there a health warning. This new exploitation of the Government's voluntary code was condemned by David

Simpson, who declared: 'This is a perfect example of why legislation is the only hope for controlling the efforts of the tobacco industry to recruit new generations of young people to its lethal and addictive product'. Philip Harris, the makers of Raffles, were forced to apologize.

On 1 August, the 20th anniversary of the ban on cigarette advertising on television, ASH wrote to the Home Secretary urging him to make the BBC and IBA observe their responsibilities under the law and to end all coverage of tobacco sponsored events.[2] ASH quoted statistics from *Marketing Magazine* showing that in 1984 British viewers saw no less than 323 hours of TV coverage of cigarette sponsored sporting events. 'The only purpose of this sponsorship is to advertise cigarettes', wrote David Simpson to the Minister. 'Not only have the tobacco companies got away with circumventing the law, they have simultaneously managed to associate their products with the very images they have promised generations of Health Ministers that they would not use in adverts, such as success in sport. Considering that cigarettes are the only consumer products that are highly dangerous when used in accordance with the manufacturers' intentions, it is amazing that society has tolerated such a flagrant breach of the law. The broadcasting authorities are as culpable as successive Governments, all for a few pieces of silver'.

In August the Health Education Council delivered a confidential submission to the Secretary of State for Social Services and the Secretary of State for the Environment calling for an end to all tobacco advertising and promotion, including sports sponsorship, by 1988. The Government-funded body told the Ministers that sponsorship of televised sport was 'making a mockery of the ban on television cigarette advertising'. There was an epidemic of smoking among children, restrictions on advertising to the young were being abused and sports sponsorship was influencing children in 'a cynical attempt to use energy, fitness and good health to promote a product that puts those "sporting" qualities at risk'.

In the submission, the chairman of the HEC, Sir Brian Bailey, replied to the argument that sport could not survive without tobacco sponsorship by pointing out that in the 13 months prior to April 1985, 216 companies new to sports sponsorship put £23.5 million into sport. His letter called for tougher and more prominent health warnings and a ban on the use of cigarette brand names for promoting adventure holidays, leisure wear and travel clubs.

Also in August Dr John Marks, chairman of the BMA Council, wrote to the Social Services Secretary, Norman Fowler, suggesting that the tobacco industry should be made more accountable for its advertising and promotional policies.[4] 'We recommend that the current negotiations should include the determination of adequate sanctions to act as a deterrent to individual companies'. In his letter Dr Marks called Mr Fowler's attention to the resolution which had been passed at the BMA's annual meeting in Plymouth and reminded him of the Department of Health's own concern as expressed in its recent direction to health authorities to clamp down on smoking. This action would be negated, he said, unless a process was started now to phase out and eventually ban the advertising and promotion of tobacco products. Dr Marks emphasized the effect which tobacco promotions had on children and young people and then turned to the issue of health warnings. 'We would like to see cigarette packets carrying a statement from the manufactuers indicating the damage that may be caused to the smoker and confirming that the manufacturer accepts responsibility for the product in the same way as any other company making and selling goods to the public. Arguments that the consumer makes a free choice of whether to smoke or not are irrelevant both in terms of consumer legislation and, more importantly, because nicotine is a highly addictive drug which the majority of people find extremely difficult to stop using once they become habituated.

Dr Marks said that in future health warnings should appear on the front and back of cigarette packets and not just on the side. The message should be changed at frequent but irregular intervals and should indicate clearly the health risks associated with the product, for example 'Smoking these (Benson and Hedges) cigarettes may cause cancer and other diseases such as chronic bronchitis'.

The BMA, still using every opportunity to get its message across to Ministers and the authorities, also submitted evidence to the Peacock committee which had been set up by the Government to consider whether the BBC should be allowed to take advertisements. In its letter the BMA expressed its concern that changes to the licence arrangements might allow further promotion of tobacco product brand names on screen. 'The view of the Independent Television Companies Association that there is no prospect of business spending more on advertising could have serious financial consequences for the BBC in the long term, particularly if Government funds are withdrawn or reduced', said the BMA. 'We do not wish to see the BBC placed in an invidious position, at risk from the tobacco and advertising industry lobbies who will argue that since tobacco goods are legal products they should be free to advertise them in any way possible'.

Throughout July and August, Pamela Taylor was holding meetings on an almost daily basis, preparing for the second phase of the campaign. She was, for instance, planning the formation of a sports group along the lines of the Artists Campaign against Tobacco Sponsorship and was in touch with several leading sports personalities. She was investigating the possibility of extending the campaign to Europe to take in the Common Market dimension, although opinion within the BMA was divided on the wisdom of this. There were plans to try and involve the trade unions, particularly women's groups within the movement, and to persuade the Labour Party to adopt an anti-smoking policy. Further parliamentary legislation was being considered and fresh approaches to the broadcasting authorities were being planned to discuss how to reduce the amount of air time being given to tobacco brand names.

As Dr John Dawson explained, 'During the first part of the campaign we explored openings to see what was going to give and what was blocked, so that in the next phase we knew where to go back and consolidate'.

There was also no doubt that the first phase of the campaign had helped create a much more hostile public image of smoking, even the introduction of a smoking ban on London's underground caused little stir. One example of this new aggression was the appearance of the country's first direct action anti-smoking groups, TREES (Those Resisting an Early End through Smoking) and its militant offshoot COFFIN came onto the scene with AGHAST (Action Group to Halt Advertising Sponsorship by Tobacco). The two organizations were an indirect result of the BMA's campaign, although neither had any connection with the Association. They were formed by a group of young doctors, mainly from the Royal Free Hospital in London, after they had attended a meeting at which Simon Chapman spoke about Australia's anti-smoking campaigns. Dr Michael Ingram, a GP trainee from Reading, had emerged as one of the organisers of TREES, whose activities included protesting at Benson and Hedges cricket matches and outside the Royal Festival Hall during a tobacco sponsored performance by the Royal Festival Ballet. COFFIN was an organization to which no one would admit belonging because its activities were strictly illegal—defacing tobacco advertising hoardings with aerosol sprays along the lines of the Australian BUGA-UP campaign.

The start of the second phase of the BMA's campaign coincided also with a ministerial reshuffle in September 1985. Mrs Thatcher promoted her two Health Ministers, Kenneth Clarke and John Patten, who left the DHSS. Mr Barney Hayhoe, a former Treasury Minister, replaced Kenneth Clarke as Health Minister and Ray Whitney, a former diplomat, moved over at the DHSS from the social security side to become junior Health Minister. As expected, the Sports Minister Neil Macfarlane left his post, having displeased the Prime Minister over his handling of the football hooliganism problem. He was replaced by a relative newcomer to Parliament, Dick Tracey, a former journalist and public relations man. These changes gave the BMA fresh opportunity to put its case to the Government on tobacco advertising and sponsorship, although even the most optimistic anti-smoking campaigners did not foresee any shift in Government policy on smoking.

The odds remained heavily stacked against the BMA. A fresh illustration of this came when Conservative MP Roger Sims had a letter published in the *Daily Telegraph* supporting the BMA's campaign. This prompted two letters to be pubished challenging Sims, who immediately wrote back in reply, but all he received was an acknowledgement from the newspaper. 'I have good reason to believe that a number of doctors wrote in supporting me', he said. 'But neither my letter nor theirs have been published, which I suppose is an editorial decision or being careful not to upset your advertisers. One just accepts this sort of thing'.

As 1985 drew to a close, all those at the BMA and its supporters in Parliament recognized that although a substantial start had been made in challenging the tobacco industry much more needed to be done if the campaign was to succeed. As Dr John Havard concluded: 'The actual achievements of the campaign will I think be shown, I hope will be shown, in a reduction or a slowing down in the increase in smoking among women. But what we have achieved is a far greater public appreciation of the dangers of smoking than was previously the case. We have had a lot of exposure and the arguments in favour of promoting the advertising of smoking have I think been remarkably unconvincing'.

REFERENCES

1. *Media Week*, July 1985.
2. DHSS press release, 31 May 1985.
3. ASH press release, 24 July 1985.
4. ASH press release, 1 August 1985.

Chapter 2

CIGARETTE ADVERTISING AND SMOKING: A REVIEW OF THE EVIDENCE

March 1985

Researched and written by
Simon Chapman, Neil Hamilton Fairley Research Fellow, National Health and Medical Research Council (Australia); Consultant, Smoking Control Programme, International Union Against Cancer (UICC), Geneva; Consultant, International Organization of Consumers' Unions (IOCU), The Hague.

SUMMARY

- All major health, medical and consumer groups have identified a ban on all forms of tobacco advertising as an essential component of a comprehensive smoking control programme.
- Tobacco advertising promotes the idea that smoking is acceptable, desirable and glamorous.
- It undermines the credibility of government health education campaigns against smoking.
- It stops the flow of full information about the health risks of smoking because many magazines and newspapers do not wish to offend their tobacco advertisers.
- If tobacco were discovered tomorrow, no government would permit its sale, let alone its advertising. The argument that legally sold products can be advertised ignores the fact that the health risks of smoking were realized long after its use had become widespread.
- Tobacco advertising redistributes the market share of different

brands and also swells demand by influencing non-smokers. Advertising by state tobacco monopolies is indisputable evidence of this.
- Children are the future of the tobacco industry and therefore primary targets for tobacco advertising. There is ample evidence of their interest in, and recall of, tobacco advertising.
- There is no evidence that tobacco advertising provides any information that encourages smokers to switch to less dangerous cigarettes.

INTRODUCTION

Cigarette advertising is the cutting-edge of the world tobacco industry's efforts to market cigarettes, a product which the World Health Organization's expert committee on smoking control described as 'responsible for more than one million premature deaths each year' worldwide[1] and control of which 'could do more to improve health and prolong life . . . than any other single action in the whole field of preventive medicine.'[2]

Smoking kills prematurely one in four men who smoke a pack or more a day. In famine-ridden countries of the developing world it competes with food for scarce arable land and the marginal survival incomes of millions of people.[3] Because of flue curing, it is thought to be responsible for one in eight of all trees felled throughout the world,[4] a problem acknowledged by the British Economist Intelligence Unit to have 'serious ecological overtones'.[5] Smoking also causes over 50 per cent of fires. Above all, the WHO expert committee on smoking control stated unequivocally: 'The international tobacco industry's irresponsible behaviour and its massive advertising and promotional campaigns are, in the opinion of the committee, direct causes of a substantial number of unnecessary deaths.'[6]

Consequently, all major international health, cancer and heart disease agencies, medical colleges and consumer organizations, notably the World Health Organization,[7-9] the World Health Assembly,[10] the International Union Against Cancer[11] and the International Organization of Consumers' Unions have agreed that all forms of tobacco promotion should be banned. In 1982, 47 countries had laws or voluntary agreements restricting certain kinds of advertising.[12] Of these, 21 (including Finland, Iceland, Italy, Norway, Senegal, Singapore, Somalia, Sudan and Yugoslavia) have banned tobacco advertising completely.

WHY BAN TOBACCO ADVERTISING?

Tobacco advertising promotes the idea that smoking is normal, good and glamorous. Tobacco advertising continually tells people that smoking is desirable. It undermines the credibility of government statements which say that smoking is bad for health. It is therefore incompatible with a government's wider smoking control policy, and leads to a widespread cynicism about health education messages. In Britain in 1983, 44 per cent of smokers questioned in a government national survey agreed that 'Smoking can't be really dangerous or the government would ban cigarette advertising.'[13] A child who grows up exposed hundreds of times a day to cigarette advertisements is less likely to accept the arguments of parents and teachers that smoking is dangerous. While the government avoids any serious restriction of tobacco promotion, its commitment to reducing smoking remains empty rhetoric.

Advertising just one factor

Tobacco advertising is not the only factor that promotes smoking. No one would argue that all a government needs to do to reduce smoking is to ban advertising. But it is of special concern because it affects other influences to smoke (like peer group and social pressures) by suggesting, for example, that a dangerous, costly, and addictive behaviour is widely held to be 'grown up', 'relaxing', 'sociable', or 'attractive'. Tobacco advertising clearly perpetuates such ideas. To argue that smoking is influenced by peer pressures at school begs the questions of where such pressures originate, and who will benefit from them.

Editorial compromise

There is also growing evidence of a further and disturbing indirect effect of cigarette advertising. Several reports[14-16] have provided strong evidence that magazines which accept tobacco advertising are less likely to publish anti-smoking articles. In one recent study, 12 large circulation US magazines were surveyed over 12 years for articles on smoking and health. Eight did not carry a single article on the hazards of smoking, despite regular articles on other health issues. Cigarette companies withdrew advertising from the *Sunday Times* after a critical article on smoking and disease named the brands smoked by the heart transplant case studies.[17] When *Newsweek* ran a story on 'the uncivil war over smoking' in June 1983, all tobacco advertisers withdrew from the magazine.[18] When four Australian state parliaments debated in 1983 whether tobacco advertising should be banned, editorial reaction was overwhelmingly negative, and many newspapers acknowledged that their guiding principle had been the money they received from advertising.[19]

Far from being the hallmark of 'freedom of expression', tobacco advertising has inhibited the flow of information on the hazards of smoking.

THE TOBACCO INDUSTRY'S PUBLIC POSITION ON ADVERTISING

Argument No. 1: 'If it's legal to sell it, it should be legal to advertise it'

This argument tries to win sympathy by portraying the tobacco industry as the victim of an anomalous and therefore unjust principle. Several points are worth making about this argument.

First, the rhetoric of the first clause ('If it is legal to sell it . . .') forces us to concede that tobacco is sold legally. The implication is that if tobacco is legal, it cannot be that bad. We now lose sight of the real issue, which is not tobacco's legal status, but its public health status as the leading cause of death in the developed world. This argument suggests that governments would be justified in outlawing advertising for an illegal product, but since tobacco is legal, an advertising ban would be incongruous. Thus, the industry tries to deflect public thinking away from considering whether promoting tobacco is in the public interest, and on to the wider issue of whether the principle should be violated, regardless of the product in question.

The argument is highly misleading. If tobacco was invented in a laboratory tomorrow, with all the information known about it available, no government would permit it to be sold. However, the health risks of tobacco were realized long after it had become widely established. If the health consequences of smoking had been known when it was introduced it is extremely doubtful that it would have become so popular, let alone been allowed to develop as an industry.

Prohibiting social drugs like alcohol and tobacco is neither feasible nor desirable, but using advertising and promotion to encourage their use is logically distinct from the issue of their legality. The argument may sound reasonable, but it is insensitive to the history of smoking, where the factors which would have influenced a decision had not yet been determined. The slogan therefore remains a convenient ruse to justify the perpetuation of tobacco advertising.

It is important to stress that tobacco is not sold freely: in Britain and in many other countries it is illegal to sell tobacco to children under 16. However all children are exposed to tobacco advertising in the same way as are adults.

'Freedom to advertise'

Hand-in-hand with this slogan is the industry's plea that it has the right to advertise its product. 'Freedom' is an emotive word carefully chosen so that the advocates of a ban can be dismissed as the enemies of freedom. But of what does this freedom really consist?

Freedom for the tobacco advertiser is the freedom to persuade people to use nicotine, an addictive drug which, having induced a strong dependency, will kill prematurely one user in four. It is quite different to the freedom experienced by most smokers, who want to stop smoking but find after many attempts that they still cannot. It is the freedom to use glossy images to distract from the fact that smoking kills and pollutes. It is the freedom to corrupt the language by calling a carcinogenic product 'mild', and using terms like 'luxury' and 'fresh' to describe it.

The 'thin end of the wedge . . .'?

A further deception is the industry's appeal: 'Where will they stop?' The industry argues that if advertising is stopped because tobacco is dangerous, then advertising for cars, motor cycles, alcohol, sugar, aircraft travel and any other potentially dangerous product could also be banned. All of these products can endanger health, but they are dangerous only when abused. Tobacco is the only advertised product which is hazardous when used as intended.

*Argument No. 2: Tobacco advertising does not influence the total demand
for tobacco, but only redistributes market share among
competing brands*

Logically, effective tobacco advertising might do four things;

- influence smokers to change brands
- influence smokers to smoke more
- influence non-smokers to start smoking
- discourage or delay smokers from giving it up.

The tobacco industry argues that it only influences smokers to change
brands. But as a writer in the trade journal Marketing noted: 'It is
curious that the only two categories of advertising that the [adver-
tising] industry suggests do not increase consumption are also those
threatened by legislation'—tobacco and alcohol.[20]

Tobacco—not a limited market

It is inconceivable that any industry would avoid trying to expand its
market. By definition, advertising seeks to maximize sales. In the few
cases where the market is limited, the function of advertising is to try
to maintain or increase brand share. However, most products have no
market ceiling, and advertising is undertaken to maintain and improve
the market share, and to expand the market. This is the case with the
tobacco industry; many people, especially children, do not smoke and
might be persuaded to take it up.

Although the industry publically denies that its advertising promotes smoking, workers in the advertising industry express contrary
views. An Australian agency executive, extending the observations of
David Abbott, a leading British advertiser, has said:

'As an argument [that tobacco advertising is only aimed at brand
switching and not at attracting new consumers] it is so preposterous it
is insulting . . . To claim that cigarette advertising does not encourage
smoking flies in the face of all advertising knowledge and experience
. . . We have the ironic situation of the Advertising Federation of
Australia, on the one hand, saying that advertising in general helps
expand markets, and thereby reduces the cost of products; and on the
other hand claiming that cigarette advertising keeps the market in a
miraculously static state.'[21]

David Abbott has said:

'I think it's incontrovertible, though people will argue against it, that advertising things encourages people to use them. The advertising industry believes that in every other product. I don't see why the rules are different for cigarettes.'[22]

And Emerson Foote, former chairman of one of the world's leading advertising agencies said about the same issue:

'This is the public position of the tobacco industry but I don't think anyone really believes this. I am not even convinced that competition among brands is the most important purpose of such advertising. I suspect that creating a positive climate of social acceptability for smoking, which encourages new smokers to join the market, is of greater importance to the industry.'[23]

Tobacco monopolies that advertise

A Rothmans executive has acknowledged that brand share is irrelevant in a monopoly situation.

'One common factor in virtually all the countries with no cigarette advertising . . . is that cigarettes are manufactured and marketed by a Government-owned and run monopoly, so the need to advertise simply does not exist.'[24]

Any advertising, therefore, must exist solely to try and increase total sales. The governments of Austria, Japan, South Korea, Thailand and Turkey have tobacco marketing monopolies, but not advertising bans.

Argument No. 3: Tobacco advertising is aimed only at adult smokers and not at children.

The Royal College of Physicians has stated: 'Learning to smoke usually occurs in childhood or in adolescence. The matter is largely settled by the age of 20; if a person is still a non-smoker at this age he is unlikely to take it up.'[25]

In Britain in 1982, children aged 11–16 spent £60 million on smoking.[26] Many young smokers maintain the habit throughout their lives

and so, from a marketing perspective, constitute the highest priority
market segment. We must assume that the tobacco industry, like all
other industries, is interested in expansion. The failure of a generation
of young people to start smoking would devastate the industry within
10 years.

Tobacco advertisements appear in media that, with the exception of
age-restricted cinema screenings, are accessible to children. Children
can see a billboard, read a newspaper or magazine, watch a television
and listen to a radio in just the way that adult smokers do. Yet the
Advertising Standards Authority's voluntary code for cigarette advertising states in its first clause that 'Cigarette advertising shall be
directed only to adult smokers and intended to effect a change of
brand.'

If the tobacco industry claims that advertisements only influence
smokers to change brands, how can these persuasive processes have
no influence on children who do not yet smoke, but who are likely to
do so soon? As a sceptical advertising industry worker wrote about
using sporting celebrities in tobacco promotions:

'. . . the cigarette industry . . . would have us believe that cigarette
advertising operates in a totally different way from every other category. That is, zeroes in on smokers and no-one else. So that when a
12-year-old boy watches the Marlboro Open, some magic barrier pre-
vents registration of the Marlboro name, but lets it through to the
smoker.'[27]

A document subpoenaed by the US Federal Trade Commission[28]
provides a rare glimpse into the advice the industry seeks and gets
from its research agencies about the approach it should take with
children.

'Thus, an attempt to reach young smokers, starters, should be based
. . . on the following major parameters:
- Present the cigarette as one of a few initiations into the adult world.
- Present the cigarette as part of the illicit pleasure category of products and activities.
- In your ads create a situation taken from the day-to-day life of the
  young smoker but in an elegant manner have this situation touch on
  the basic symbols of the growing-up, maturity process.
- To the best of your ability (considering some legal restraints) relate
  the cigarette to 'pot', wine, beer, sex, etc.
- DON'T communicate health or health-related points.'

The industry makes great play of studies which ask children to say whether they think they are influenced by advertisements. Children, like adults, report that they are not, and that friends and parents influence them to smoke. Such studies are methodologically unsound: there is a world of difference in believing that one is not influenced by advertising, and whether in fact one is influenced. Similar results are found for all sorts of products: people seldom admit to, or are aware of, the influence of advertising. Bergler, in a book much favoured by the advertising industry, states that any self-report about the influence of advertising on smoking or brand choice is 'quite worthless'.[29]

However, some research has provided legitimate and important information about children and tobacco advertising. Three recent Australian studies have provided highly indicative data. The first, a study of children's beliefs about the general intentions and effects of cigarette advertising,[30] found that:

- over 80 per cent believed that advertisements probably encourage children to take up smoking.
- 36 per cent said that children liked cigarette advertisements.
- 74 per cent said that advertisements try to make smoking look healthy.
- 73 per cent said that advertisements try to make smoking seem better than not smoking.

A study of 5686 children found that 'approval of cigarette advertising' was second only to having friends who smoked as the best predictor of whether a child would subsequently smoke.[31] Students were questioned twice, with a year in between, and those who had approved of cigarette advertising were twice as likely to have become smokers as those who had disapproved.[32] Former non-smoking disapprovers of cigarette advertising who had started to smoke had also changed their attitudes to cigarette advertising.

A third study[33] found that adolescent smokers select heavily advertised brands at up to twice the rate of adult smokers, and that children who smoke are twice as likely as non-smokers to recognize cigarette advertisements and slogans. Finally, a 1984 British survey of 880 children found that children are most aware of brands most frequently associated with televised sporting events, and that awareness of one brand increased following a major snooker tournament sponsored by that brand.[34]

*Argument No. 4:   Cigarette advertising provides smokers with 'information'
which persuades them to convert to 'safer' filtered and
low-tar cigarettes. Advertising bans are therefore inimical
to both freedom of information and to public health.*

Few categories of advertising can provide consumers with so little
information as cigarette advertising. What information is provided by
the Marlboro man, by the slashed silk in Silk Cut advertisements, or
by the cryptic Benson and Hedges series? The argument over information on tar content can easily be met by the suggestion that all
cigarette sellers be required to display a tar table, a simple solution
that the tobacco industry has nowhere implemented. In Finland,
where tobacco advertising is banned, dramatic reductions in tar content have been achieved through government directives to the industry.

However, Waterson,[35] in a booklet on advertising and smoking produced by the British Advertising Association and distributed widely by
the tobacco industry, argues that 'it is obvious . . . that an advertising
ban slows down the rate of conversion of smokers from plain to filtered cigarettes' and 'from high-tar to low tar products'. He has two
tables comparing nations with and without advertising bans to support his claim. He shows five countries with advertising bans where
more than 30 per cent of smokers smoke non-filter cigarettes, and
nine that do allow advertising, where less than 10 per cent smoke
non-filter brands. He apparently selected these because there was
high filtered cigarette consumption, which contrasted for polemical
purposes with an equally selective group without advertising. He
could have constructed a table for the same year showing countries
which allowed advertising but also had high non-filter consumption:
for example Mexico (more than 80 per cent); India (more than 61 per
cent); Pakistan (more than 57 per cent); and Netherlands (more than 28
per cent).[36] This would have produced a totally different result.

THE EVIDENCE OF CIGARETTE
ADVERTISING'S INFLUENCE

So far the case against tobacco advertising has been stated in common-
sense terms: tobacco advertising and promotion, as the words

suggest, advertise and promote cigarettes. One cannot promote cigarettes without implicitly promoting smoking, so the industry's argument that its advertising is only solely concerned with brand promotion is specious.

As early as the 1940s, researchers were forthright about the effects of tobacco advertising. Borden, professor of advertising at Harvard, concluded that advertising was an important factor in determining both the size and speed of consumption . . . 'Without advertising cigarette use would probably have grown; with advertising, the increase has been amazing.'[37]

The Metra study

The industry has widely promoted the Metra study,[38] which it funded, and which concluded that advertising did not expand the total market for tobacco. It was based on data supplied by the industry which have not been published because of alleged confidentiality.[39] The following criticisms, among many others, can be made of the report.[40]

1. It assumes that advertising immediately affects consumption, whereas the relationship is far more oblique:

   'Advertising is often considered to be of an investment nature, building up a fund of goodwill towards products that slowly decays in the absence of advertising, but still yields influence. If the marginal effects of additional advertising to this fund are small and if it decays at a low rate, then changes in advertising between two years will have only a little influence on behaviour and it will only be possible to see the effects in the long run.'[41]

2. It ignored children's smoking completely. Since adult smoking rates have declined significantly recently and teenage rates have increased, such analysis is essential.
3. It ignored the likely effects of the increasing anti-smoking publicity, the increasing use of sponsorship, and the increasing number of no-smoking areas in public spaces.

AS WAS EXPECTED . . . THE INDUSTRY'S OWN DATA

The most recently published study on the subject is that of Reuijl,[42] funded partly by West German tobacco companies, which examined cigarette and advertising data in that country between 1961 and 1975. The companies provided 'highly confidential figures'. Reuijl concluded that advertising had a 'highly significant influence on primary demand' (i.e. on total industry sales) and that this was an 'obvious counter-example . . . for the hypothesis that saturated markets are characterized by reciprocal cancellation of brand advertising.' In other words, advertising did not just influence existing smokers, but also increased the total number of people smoking. Not surprisingly, the industry has not publicized this study, although it is the most recent and the most authoritative yet.

THE ADVERTISING BAN IN NORWAY

In 1970, the Norwegian parliament decided to introduce a smoking control programme that included health education in schools, warnings on cigarette packets and a ban on all tobacco advertising and promotion. The Norwegian Tobacco Act came into force in July 1975. Official figures from the Norwegian customs and excise show that cigarette sales declined markedly at the time of the 1970 announcement and also after the Act came into force (see Figure 1).

The Norwegian programme and legislation is considered to be the outstanding model by international smoking control agencies and its correspondence with the declines in smoking has often been cited as evidence that advertising bans affect tobacco consumption, a relationship which the tobacco and advertising industries have often disputed. Neither side disputes that cigarette smoking decreased, but while health groups said that it was caused by the ban on advertising, the industry argued that the falls began before the advertising ban. However, it is indisputable that the introduction of the ban in 1975 was associated with a further decline in smoking. Norwegian children who had been smoking more before the ban, smoked fewer cigarettes after its introduction (see Figure 2).

The announcement in 1970 of a major programme on smoking and health generated considerable interest throughout Norway. As the

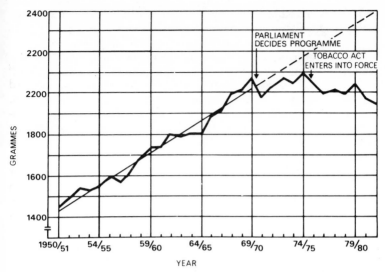

FIGURE 1   Sales of smoking tobacco and manufactured cigarettes *per capita*, age 15 years +, 1950/51 to 1981/82 in Norway.

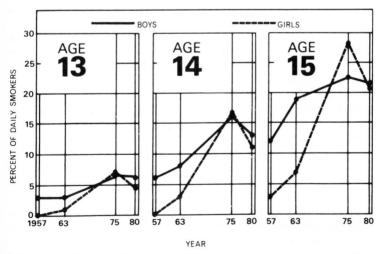

FIGURE 2   Percentage of daily smokers among Norwegian school pupils aged 13–15 years, 1957 to 1982.

broken line in Figure 1 indicates, if the trend in *per capita* consumption prior to 1970 had continued, consumption would have been 23 per cent higher than actually occurred in 1981/2 had the trend in consumption before 1970 continued. The unprecedented downturn may well be explained by a synergism between the measures introduced after 1970 and the heightened community awareness. Alternatively, single measures such as the advertising ban may have been the key factor. For reasons described below, it is impossible to assess the impact of specific variables without sacrificing methodological rigour.

IMPOSSIBILITY OF ISOLATING THE PRECISE EFFECT OF ADVERTISING

The tobacco industry always insists that those who advocate a ban on advertising must come up with hard evidence that it influences consumption, yet they know that the exact influence of tobacco advertising cannot be assessed. As a current Rothman's executive has stated:

'This (claim that cigarette advertising reinforces the act of cigarette smoking and hence increases total consumption to a level beyond what it might have been in the absence of advertising) is particularly difficult to refute as the only true test would be to study the consumption trend in a number of different markets under conditions of full cigarette advertising and no cigarette advertising, but over the same period as to achieve identical economical and social pressures. This is clearly impossible.'[43]

Tobacco advertising is only one factor influencing the decision to smoke; others include social, religious, parental, sibling and peer smoking behaviour and attitudes, price and disposable income, age limit proscriptions, intelligence and social class. To isolate the effect of one factor would mean holding the others constant. These factors are different from country to country, continually changing.

Yet, in the public debate, the industry often characterizes as comparable quite diverse countries on the basis that they have no tobacco advertising, thereby obscuring often crucial differences in social climates and government positions on smoking. By the industry's argument, an Eastern bloc country with no advertising and increasing numbers of smokers is evidence that banning advertising will not slow a country's smoking rate. They do not refer to any other factors. But, for example, the Soviet Union, often cited by the industry as an example without advertising but with widespread smoking, has the cheapest tobacco and a virtual absence of any smoking control measures.[44] The rise in consumption could be much steeper if advertising were added to those factors already forcing up consumption.

Effect of partial bans

The industry also argues that partial advertising bans have not worked. But in countries where tobacco advertising is banned from radio and television, such as Australia, the UK and the USA, massive amounts of advertising expenditure have been transferred into other media such as print, outdoor events and sponsorship. Partial bans can be expected to have only partial effects.

SPORTING AND CULTURAL SPONSORSHIP

So-called indirect or incidental tobacco advertising is most common in countries where direct tobacco advertising is banned from radio and television. During the 1981/2 Australian cricket season, the sponsor, Benson and Hedges, received what was described as 'a stupefying 40,000 exposures' on one TV channel alone 'ranging from quick flashes to long, languid camera pans of their distinctive, strategically-placed 300 metres of ground level hoarding'.[45] In Britain in 1983, more than 327 hours of tobacco-sponsored events were screened on television.[46]

Advertising through sporting and cultural sponsorship has three main advantages for the tobacco industry. First, such advertising is not usually classified as advertising, and therefore can circumvent advertising bans to the extent that more tobacco advertising is seen on television than would otherwise occur. Second, sponsorship tends to build a constituency of thankful and financially dependent recipients who can often be relied on to support the industry.

Finally, and perhaps most obviously, sponsorship associates sporting prowess and cultural excellence with cigarettes in ways that self-regulated codes of conduct forbid. For example, the British Code of Advertising Practice's voluntary code on tobacco states that 'advertisements should not imply that smoking is associated with success in

sport. They should not depict people participating in any active sporting pursuit or obviously about to do so or just having done so, or
spectators at any organized sporting occasion.'

Such associations tend to insulate the industry against criticism
whereby 'adversaries must implicitly criticize these values in order to
raise objections to the ad message.'[47] Criticizing a sporting hero for
taking tobacco money will be seen by many as 'unsporting'. Like any
other sponsor, tobacco companies can give money anonymously; that
they choose not to do so, must be seen in terms of their desire to
associate their product with popular and prestigious events.

The tobacco industry knows well the value of such exposure. The
chairman, president and chief executive reporter of RJ Reynolds
Tobacco Co. told the Tobacco Reporter about its sponsorship of horse
racing 'We made it clear from the day we announced our sponsorship
of the Grand National Division that we were in the business of selling
cigarettes, not the racing business.'[48] Rod Marsh, the Australian test
cricketer, has said that the value Benson and Hedges received from
their cricket sponsorship 'was absolutely bloody ridiculous. They
were laughing all the way to the bank.'[49] Companies like MacDonalds,
who sponsor cricket in Australia, make no bones about their desire to
attract children to their product. Why should we believe tobacco's
sponsorship of sport has any other motives?

CONCLUSION

The bottom line in all argument about alleged freedoms, the role of
the state, and tobacco advertising is the appalling, unnecessary and
totally avoidable health consequences of smoking. Those who believe
that the epidemic of premature smokers' deaths matters less than the
corporate health of the tobacco industry will doubtless be long
remembered in the history of public health. Others have different
priorities, and have equally direct arguments to oppose tobacco
advertising. They need say no more than the obvious truth that
tobacco promotions seek to, and inevitably often succeed in, promoting smoking, which kills more than one million people worldwide
each year. If arguments remain to delay legislation banning tobacco
advertising, they will have nothing to do with public health.

ACKNOWLEDGEMENTS

For their critical comments and suggestions: Mike Daube, Charles Fletcher, Bobbie Jacobson, David Simpson and Patti White.

REFERENCES

1. World Health Organization. Smoking control strategies in developing countries. *Technical Report Series 695*, World Health Organization, Geneva, 1983, p. 8.
2. World Health Organization. Report of a WHO Expert Committee. Smoking and its effects on health. *Technical Report Series 568*. World Health Organization, Geneva, 1975, p. 8.
3. Cohen, N. Smoking, health and survival: prospects of Bangladesh. *Lancet*, 1981, 1090–93.
4. Madeley, J. The environmental impact of tobacco production in developing countries. *New York State Journal of Medicine*, 1983, 83, 1310–11.
5. Economist Intelligence Unit Limited. *Leaf tobacco: its contribution to the economic and social development of the Third World*, EIU, London; 1980.
6. World Health Organization. Report of the WHO Expert Committee on Smoking Control. Controlling the Smoking Epidemic. *Technical Report Series 636*, World Health Organization, Geneva; 1979, p. 9.
7. World Health Organization, Reference 2.
8. World Health Organization, Reference 6.
9. World Health Organization, Reference 1.
10. World Health Assembly. *Resolutions of the 33rd World Health Assembly*, Geneva, 1980, May 23.
11. Gray, N. and Daube, M. Guidelines for smoking control. *Technical Report Series Vol. 52*, 2nd Edition, Union International Contre Le Cancer (U.I.C.C.), Geneva.
12. Roemer, R. *Legislative action to combat the world smoking epidemic*. World Health Organization, Geneva, 1982.
13. Marsh, A. and Matheson, J. *Smoking attitudes and behaviour*. An enquiry carried out on behalf of the Department of Health and Social Security. Office of Population Censuses and Surveys. HMSO, London, 1983.
14. Whelan, E. M. *et al.* Analysis of coverage of tobacco hazards in women's magazines, *Journal of Public Health Policy*, 1981, March, 28–35.
15. Smith, R. C. The magazines' smoking habit. *Columbia Journalism Review*, 1978, Jan/Feb, 29–31.
16. Whelan, E. M. When Newsweek and Time filtered cigarette copy. *The Wall Street Journal*, 1984, Nov. 1.
17. Hird, C. Taking on the tobacco men. *New Statesman*, 1981, Feb. 27.
18. Anon. Tobacco ads withdrawn. *Advertising News*, 1983, Jul. 1.
19. Chapman, S. Not biting the hand that feeds you. Tobacco advertising and editorial bias in Australian newspapers. *Medical Journal of Australia*, 1984, 140, 480–2.

20. Barnett, B. On the links between bulls and cigarettes. *Marketing (U.K.)*, 1983, Mar. 10, p. 7.
21. Dumas, A. Cigarette ads—conscience versus profits. *Broadcasting and Television Weekly*. 1978, Aug. 10.
22. Daube, M. Towards an advertising ban. *Proceedings of the 3rd World Conference on Smoking and Health*. Public Health Service, US DHEW, National Institute of Health DHEW Pub. no. (NIH) 77–1413, 1975.
23. Foote, E. Advertising and tobacco. *Journal of the American Medical Association*, 1981, **245**, 1667–68.
24. Ryan, W. P. (Rothmans) Cigarette advertising—Its role and rationale. Paper presented to Health Advisory Council, Health Commission of NSW, 1978, Jul. 17.
25. Royal College of Physicians of London. *Smoking or health. The third report of the Royal College of Physicians of London*. Pitman Medical, London, 1978, p. 104.
26. Dobbs, J. and Marsh, A. *Smoking among secondary school children*. Office of Population Censuses and Surveys. Social Survey Division. HMSO, London, 1983.
27. Dumas, A. Reference 21.
28. Federal Trade Commission Staff Report on the Cigarette Advertising Investigation. Chapter 2, footnote 40. Document A901268 May 26, 1975 'What have we learned from people? A conceptual summarization of 18 focus group interviews on the subject of smoking.'
29. Bergler, R. *Advertising and cigarette smoking*. Hans Huber, Bern, 1981.
30. Fisher, D. A. and Magnus, P. Out of the mouths of babes . . . the opinions of 10 year old and 11 year old children regarding the advertising of cigarettes. *Community Health Studies*, 1981, **5**(1), 22–26.
31. O'Connell, D. L. *et al*. Cigarette smoking and drug use in schoolchildren. II factors associated with smoking. *International Journal of Epidemiology*, 1981, **10**(3), 223–31.
32. Alexander, H. M. *et al*. Cigarette smoking and drug use in schoolchildren: IV—factors associated with changes in smoking behaviour. *International Journal of Epidemiology*, 1983, **12**(1), 59–66.
33. Chapman, S. and Fitzgerald, B. Brand preference and advertising recall in adolescent smokers: some implications for health promotion. *American Journal of Public Health*, 1982, **73**, 491–4.
34. Ledwith, F. Does tobacco sports sponsorship on television act as advertising to children? *Health Education Journal*, 1984, **43**(4), 85–8.
35. Waterson, M. J. *Advertising and cigarette consumption*. The Advertising Association, London, Fourth Edition, 1983, Sep. p. 7.
36. Maxwell, J. S. How the brands ranked. Maxwell international estimates. Published annually in World Tobacco.
37. Borden, N. H. The economic effects of advertising. Richard D. Irwin, Chicago, 1942, 227–8.
38. Sinnot, P. R. J, Gillian, R. J. and Kyle, P. W. The relationship between total cigarette advertising and total cigarette consumption in the U.K. Volumes 1 and 2. METRA Consulting Group, London, 1979, Oct.
39. McGuinness, A. J. Cigarette advertising (letter). *Financial Times* (U.K.) 1980, Jun. 5.
40. Fletcher, C. M. *Critique of the METRA Report. Action on Smoking and Health*. Note of ASH criticisms of tobacco industry's METRA Report. Press release, 1980, Jan. 15.

41. Wickstrom, B. Cigarette marketing in the Third World. A study of four countries. University of Gothenburg Department of Business Administration, 1979.
42. Reuijl, J. C. *On the determination of advertising effectiveness: an empirical study of the German cigarette market*. Boston, Kluwer-Nijhoff, 1982, p. 81.
43. Government of Western Australia. Committee on the Monitoring of the Advertising of Tobacco Products. Interim Report for the Minister of Health, 1980, Jul.
44. Staroselsky, L. A poison industry? *Tobacco Reporter*, 1981, April, 46–7.
45. Summer, J. Sponsors the real winners from cricket's big scores. *Sydney Morning Herald*, 1982, Feb. 9, p. 7.
46. Etherington, R. *Sportscan* (UK) 1983.
47. Sethi, S. P. *Advocacy advertising and large corporations*. Lexington Books, Lexington, Mass. 1977, p. 17.
48. Anon. Can television be replaced? *Tobacco Reporter*. 1980, Aug., 21–5.
49. Butler, K. *Howzat*. Collins, Sydney, 1979, 86.

Chapter 3

WHEN SMOKE GETS IN YOUR EYES CIGARETTE ADVERTISING POLICY AND COVERAGE OF SMOKING AND HEALTH IN WOMEN'S MAGAZINES

May 1985

Bobbie Jacobson, Research Fellow in Health Promotion, London School of Hygiene and Tropical Medicine; Author of 'The Ladykillers—Why Smoking is a Feminist Issue'.

Amanda Amos, Senior Scientific Officer, Departments of Health Education and Community Medicine, Hampstead Health Authority, London.

THE BATTLEFIELD

Increasing concern about the rising female death toll from cigarette smoking, the slower decline of smoking among women and the rising proportion of girls smoking prompted this survey of cigarette advertising and health coverage on smoking in 53 British women's magazines. Read by over half of all British women, they form an under-recognized battlefield for pro- and anti-smoking forces. The results are summarized below.

Cigarette Advertising and General Advertising Policies

'I am positively against smoking or any encouragement of it, and wish my company would turn down cigarette advertising' Editor, *Good Housekeeping*.

- 64 per cent of the magazines in this study accepted cigarette advertisements. In contrast a recent Government-commissioned opinion
poll found that over half the women questioned were in favour of a
ban on cigarette advertising in newspapers and magazines.

'We don't accept advertisements for products known or suspected to
be hazardous to health' Managing Editor, *Just Seventeen*.

- All but two of the magazines which responded operated a clear
policy of screening advertisements for their acceptibility. Most
rejected certain products on the grounds that they were either
'hazardous', 'offensive', 'misleading', 'anti-female', 'unaesthetic' or
'inappropriate'. Yet nearly two-thirds accepted cigarette advertising
which represented an average of 7 per cent of total advertising
revenue, and ranged from less than 1 per cent to 14 per cent for
each magazine.

'Although a firm believer in anti-smoking, it isn't always possible to
turn down the kind of lucrative advertising the tobacco industry generates' Editor, *Ms London*.

- Revenue was cited as the most important reason for accepting
cigarette advertising, yet 93 per cent of the magazines' revenue in
this study came from non-tobacco sources. And contrary to the
widely held belief that magazines cannot exist without cigarette
advertising revenue, 32 per cent of the sample refused cigarette
advertising, and many of these were clearly thriving. Indeed previous research has shown that newspapers and magazines are not
only prepared to replace revenue lost from tobacco with other
sources but have been successful in doing so.

Cigarette Advertising and Young Readers

'Being very anti-smoking I would never take on any advertising for
cigarettes' Editor, *Loving*.

- It is declared Government policy that young people should not be
exposed to cigarette advertising. This principle of practice is
embodied in the Advertising Standards Authority's (ASA) Code of
Advertising Practice on cigarette advertising. The essence of this

code is that 'Advertisements should not seek to encourage people, particularly the young to start smoking'; and Rule 2.12. precludes cigarette advertisements appearing in any publication directed wholly or mainly to young people.

- Nearly two thirds of magazines with a majority of readers aged 15–24 accepted cigarette advertising, and 93 per cent of magazines whose numerically largest readership group was aged 15–24, also accepted cigarette advertisements. This represents a total of 58 per cent of magazines with a predominantly under 25 readership profile which accepted cigarette advertising.

- A separate analysis of 14 magazines read mainly by teenagers and young women showed that half accepted cigarette advertising, and that in more than half of these, the proportion of female readers aged 15–19 was greater than those aged 20–24. Extrapolating from these magazines alone, at least 1.2 million teenage girls are exposed to cigarette advertising. Of these readers aged 15–19 who smoked, most are still experimental smokers, and therefore highly vulnerable to cigarette advertising. In over half the magazines which accepted cigarette advertising, smoking rates were above 40 per cent—much higher than the average 30 per cent for 15–19 year olds in general.

- The majority of young readers in all cases were still non-smokers. The high rate of acceptance of cigarette advertising in magazines read by teenagers and young women means that at least 1 million non-smokers aged 15–24 are being exposed to cigarette advertising. These results clearly show that the tobacco companies are in breach not only of their Voluntary Agreement with Government but also the ASA code on cigarette advertising.

Smoking and Health Coverage

'The difficulty is that we take money from these people. . . . It does not matter how much we take from them it's difficult for us to endorse anything that goes against the companies. Even editorially, they have to go carefully. The tobacco companies are very sensitive about their image' Advertising Department, *Woman*.

• Evidence from the USA, Australia and the UK clearly shows that the acceptance of cigarette advertising has resulted in either the de-emphasis or removal altogether of editorial references to the effects of smoking on health. This study shows that only 37 per cent of British magazines had recently given or were planning to give major coverage to the topic. Those most heavily dependent on revenue from cigarettes were less likely to have covered the topic, but some magazines which accepted cigarette advertising had also given good coverage to smoking and health. In all these magazines the number of pages devoted to smoking and health was always over-whelmingly outweighed by the number of cigarette advertisements.

'We are very sympathic to the issue and are very committed to its serious coverage' Health Editor, *Vogue*.

'We tend not to cover it as a major issue. We assume our readers know all about the risks' Editor, *Woman's World*.

• A key factor in determining the amount of coverage given to smoking and health was the personal interest and commitment of the editor. However, coverage was disappointinly low in most young teenage magazines, many of whose readers are under maximum pressure to start smoking.

RECOMMENDATIONS

To Government

1. There should be legislation to ban all tobacco advertising and promotion.
2. In the interim the ASA code should be strengthened so that it is not possible to advertise cigarettes in youth magazines, and this should be defined as any magazines whose largest readership group is under 25.
3. The tobacco industry should be instructed to stop breaking its voluntary agreement with the Government, and cease advertising in youth magazines forthwith.

To the Tobacco Industry

1. It should cease advertising forthwith in magazines with predominantly young readers.

To Magazines and Editorial Staff

1. All magazines with a predominantly youthful profile should stop all cigarette advertising.
2. Dependency on cigarette advertising in all magazines should be reduced, with the eventual aim of stopping altogether.
3. Regular coverage should be given to aspects of smoking including health, giving up smoking and non-smokers' rights.
4. Teenage and youth magazines should make special efforts to increase awareness of the special risks that smoking poses to young women, such as smoking and the pill and smoking in pregnancy.
5. Magazines should avoid, where possible, using glamorous pictures of people smoking.

To Health Educators and Health Professionals

1. Better contacts with editorial staff should be forged so that a more regular exchange of information on this topic can take place.
2. The issue of cigarette advertising should be raised personally with editors, or through the letters pages or the Advertising Standards Authority in case of breaches of its cigarette advertising code.

To Readers and The General Public

1. Breaches of the ASA's cigarette advertising code can be raised with magazine editors, the ASA, local MPs and the Government.
2. Concerns about any aspect of smoking can be raised with magazines themselves.

INTRODUCTION

Increasing attention is now being focused on the growing intensity of
the smoking problem among girls and women.[1] Ten years ago, most
research into smoking prevalence among teenagers showed that more
boys than girls were smokers.[2,3] By the end of the decade this pattern
had changed, and in 1982 smoking rates for girls and boys were equal
in most age groups.[4] In a number of recent studies, the proportion of
girls smoking in their mid-teens has now overtaken boys.[5–8]
Moreover, anti-smoking campaigns appear to have had more effect on
adult men than women, and smoking is declining much faster in men
than women. Between 1972 and 1982 smoking declined by 27 per cent
in men but only by 20 per cent in women. The large gap that used to
exist between the percentage of men and women smokers is now
closed in most younger age groups, and in 1982 the overall percentage
of women smoking (33 per cent) lagged only 5 per cent behind men,
38 per cent of whom smoked.[9] There are proportionately fewer
women ex-smokers in every social class and age group except the
youngest,[10] and a growing body of evidence shows that women find it
harder to stop smoking than men.[11]

The burgeoning female death toll from smoking-induced
disease—which killed nearly 33,000 British women in 1983[12] from
coronary heart disease, lung cancer and chronic bronchitis—reflects
the large-scale growth of smoking among women since the last World
War. While lung cancer is now declining among men, it is rising inexorably among women, and has already overtaken breast cancer as the
biggest cause of death from cancer in women aged between 65 and
74.[13] Smoking also imposes unique, increased risks for young
women. Those who take the contraceptive pill and smoke have an
increased risk of coronary heart disease and stroke (mainly subarachnoid haemorrhage).[14] New evidence has also linked smoking to cancer
of the cervix.[15] Smoking is also known to harm the unborn baby[16] and
is linked to an earlier menopause.[17]

In the face of these problems the tobacco industry, which spends at
least £100 million on its promotions, has increasingly targeted both its
product and its advertising at women. Indeed a leading tobacco trade
journal has openly stated that 'Women are a prime target as far as any
alert European marketing man is concerned.'[18]

The potential of women's magazines as a medium for promoting smoking on the one hand, and informing women about smoking and health on the other, has largely been ignored by health educators. In contrast, tobacco companies are well aware of the importance of this medium as a way of reaching women. In recent years they have proved to be an ideal medium for launching brands such as *Virginia Slims* and *Kim* which were aimed exclusively at young women. The audience for these magazines is massive, and they are read regularly by over half of women in Britain.[19] They reach women of all ages and all social backgrounds, and many, particularly the glossy monthlies, also have the advantage of a long 'stayability' effect. As they can lie around on view for up to several months after publication, they there-fore have a readership which can be many times higher than their circulation. With these advantages in mind, it is not surprising that women's magazines have today become one of the more important media outlets for cigarette advertising. Between 1977 and 1982 revenue from tobacco advertising in women's magazines increased from £2.4 to £4.5 million. Adjusted for inflation, this represented a real increase of nearly 50 per cent.[20] As a result women's magazines in general have become more reliant on cigarette advertisements as a source of revenue. By 1984, their total earnings from cigarettes had reached £6.9 million.[21]

Women's magazines have a long tradition of acting as sources of information and advice on a wide range of topics including health.[22,23] It is widely believed that because of the closeness of the relationship between these magazines and their readers, that may have developed over many years, women are more likely to trust and value the infor-mation offered by these magazines compared with other media.[24] Both editorial staff and readers see women's magazines as a major source of information about health. An analysis of five major women's magazines in 1982 showed that 9–13 per cent of editorial pages were devoted to health topics. Its conclusion was that all but one magazine 'regarded health as an important, relevant and appropriate subject for their magazine to cover'.[25] A survey of over 200 people in pre-retirement groups found that 81 per cent claimed that they obtained most of their information about nutrition from magazines and news-papers.[26]

Women's magazines clearly have an important agenda-setting role in defining ideas about health and the causes of ill-health.[27] Because they provide a large, attentive audience that is open to both pro- and anti-health forces, we chose to survey their policies on cigarette advertising and editorial coverage of smoking and health.

METHODS

We surveyed 53 magazines between August 1984 and February 1985. All had a predominantly female readership, usually 75 per cent or more. Most were overtly geared to women, but in our efforts to cover major magazines read by young women, we also included three magazines (*Smash Hits*, *The Face* and *No 1*) which were not specifically aimed at women, but had a large, young female readership.

The editor of each magazine was sent a letter asking for the following information:

1. A copy of the most recent article on smoking and health published in the magazine.
2. The size of the magazine's readership and the age range of the target readership.
3. The magazine's policy on advertising in general and cigarettes in particular, and what proportion, if any, of the total advertising revenue came from cigarettes.
4. The Editor's views on the effect of cigarette advertising directed at women.

Non-respondents were sent a further identical letter with a covering note, followed up with a phone call to the editor. Final non-respondents were defined as those who had neither responded to the letters nor up to four follow up phone calls to the editor. Where editors were not able to answer all the questions missing information was recorded in a separate phone call to advertising departments, and health editors. In one case, IPC, it was necessary to confirm advertising policy in youth magazines with the Group Advertising Controller for Youth Magazines.

We took a general policy on advertising to mean any policy in which a product or products had been, or were likely to be refused. All magazines which did not accept cigarette advertisements, were regarded, by definition, as operating a general advertising policy. We took acceptance of cigarette advertising to mean acceptance or preparedness to accept any cigarette advertisements at any time. Estimates for revenue from cigarette advertising were based on what editors or advertising departments said—whichever was higher. Where no clear information on revenue was available, an estimate was calculated for each magazine. This was based on the proportion of full page advertisement equivalents taken as an average of two or more separate issues between June 1984 and February 1985. This was, necessarily, an underestimate because cigarette advertisements are usually placed in prime sites.

We recorded all major articles on smoking and health sent to us, and any clear references to planned, future articles by the editor as positive coverage of smoking and health. All references by editors to 'possible' articles and 'probable' past coverage of the issue were excluded. We divided the magazines' responses into four groups according to the predominant age of their readership.

RESULTS

General Advertising Policy

Forty-six out of 53 (87 per cent) magazines responded. Tables 1–4 show that all but two of the magazines which replied—*Over 21* and *House and Garden*—operated a discriminatory or screening policy on advertising in general. Most magazines mentioned rejecting individual advertisements or certain product groups—usually on the grounds that they were either 'hazardous', 'offensive', 'misleading', 'anti-female', 'unaesthetic', or 'inappropriate' to the image of the magazine. Magazines which rejected certain products on health grounds tended to be those which rejected cigarettes for the same reasons. These were mostly young teenage magazines (Table 1), health/fitness magazines and those devoted to parentcraft and children. For example, *No 1* refused advertisements for alcohol as well as cigarettes, *New Health* would not accept any product known to be hazardous to health, neither would *Just Seventeen* or *My Guy*. *Parents* rejected all alcohol, sugar and confectionary products as well as tobacco. Many of the magazines which accepted cigarette advertisements also mentioned rejecting other products on health grounds. *Woman's Own* has turned down advertising for vaginal deodorants. *Vogue* and *Harpers and Queen* have refused health clinic advertisements which made spurious claims. Similarly, *The Lady* has refused some advertisements for nursing homes. Charlotte Lessing, editor of *Good Housekeeping*, sometimes turns down advertisements in the 'medical and beauty' line which, she said, 'slip through the net of the Advertising Standards Authority, but which we prefer not to accept because we disagree, disapprove or feel they could be harmful to

TABLE 1 Young teenage magazines—where the majority of readers were under 19

Magazine	Total female readership[a] (000s)	General advertising policy	Acceptance of cigarette advertising	Smoking and health coverage (recent major articles)	Publisher
Blue Jeans	515	Yes	No	No	IPC
Jackie	813	Yes	No	Yes	D. C. Thomson
Just 17	600[b]	Yes	No	Yes[c]	EMAP
My Guy	547	Yes	No	No	IPC
No 1	1000[b]	Yes	No	No	IPC
Oh Boy	337	Yes	No	Magazine closed down Jan 1985	IPC
Patches	387	Yes	No	No	IPC
Smash Hits	1,200[b]	Yes	No	No	EMAP

[a]Estimates for readership are from National Readership Survey (NRS) figures Jan–June 1984.
[b]NRS figures not available. Estimate from magazine itself.
[c]See Reference 28.

TABLE 2 Older teenage and younger women's magazines—where the majority of readers were 15–24

Magazine	Female readership[a]		Target reader's age (magazine's view)	General advertising policy	Acceptance of cigarette advertising	Revenue from cigarette ads	Publisher
	Total (000s)	% 15–24					
Company	788	55	20s	Yes	Yes	14%[b]	National Magazines
Girls About Town	250	53	17–34	Yes	Yes	Very low	GAT Magazine Ltd
Honey	598	56	—	—	Yes	3%[b]	IPC
Look Now	532	79	18–21	No	No	None	Carlton
Loving	295	69	16–24	Yes	No	None	IPC
Ms London	287	54	15–34	Yes	Yes	Very low	Employment Publishing Ltd
19	546	73	15–30	Yes	No	None	IPC
Over 21	722	63	—	No	Yes	13%[b]	M S Publishing

[a] Estimates for readership are from National Readership Survey (NRS) figures Jan–June 1984.
[b] Calculated estimate.

TABLE 3 Younger women's magazines—where the numerically largest readership group was 15–24

Magazine	Female readership[a]		Target reader's age (magazine's view)	General advertising policy	Acceptance of cigarette advertising	Revenue from cigarette ads	Publisher
	Total (000s)	% 15–24					
Annabel	812	25	—	Yes	Yes	10%[d]	D. C. Thomson
Cosmopolitan	1866	45	—	Yes	Yes	5%	National Magazines
Fitness	100[b,c]	—	18–35	Yes	No	None	Stonehart Leisure
Harpers & Queen	573	22	30–40	Yes	Yes	4%[d]	National Magazines
Mother & Baby	726	38	—	—	—	—	Argus
Options	845	40	20–40	Yes	Yes	'Small' 5%[d]	Carlton

She	1167	26	25–44	Yes	Yes	8%	National Magazines
Slimming	1332	34	No average reader	Yes	Yes	'Occasionally' 2%[d]	SM Publications Ltd
The Face	67[c]	—	18–30	Yes	Yes	Only 1 ever published	Wagadon Ltd
True Romances	1294	38	18–24	Yes	Yes	10%	Argus
True Story	836	31	16–34	Yes	Yes	10%	Argus
Vogue	1652	40	A broad age spread	Yes	Yes	3%	Conde Nast
Woman	3846	25	25–44	Yes	Yes	9%[e]	IPC
Woman's Own	4641	24	25–35	Yes	Yes	8%[e]	IPC
Woman's World	1049	33	25–40	Yes	Yes	7%	Carlton

[a]Estimates for readership are from National Readership Survey (NRS) figures Jan–June 1984.
[b]Because of its recent launch, there is no full readership breakdown for Fitness. An analysis in Campaign (The Battle to Survive/in the Health War, Richard Eyre, May 4, 1984, pp 43–51) showed most ABC1 buyers to be aged 15–24.
[c]Circulation figure from magazine, readership figures not yet available.
[d]Calculated estimate.
[e]IPC unpublished.

TABLE 4   Older women's magazines where the majority of readers were over 25

Magazine	Female readership[a] (000s)	General advertising policy	Acceptance of cigarette advertising	Revenue from cigarette ads	Publisher
Family Circle	2708	Yes	Yes	4%	International Thomson Publ
Fashioncraft	—	—	—	—	Litharne Ltd
Good Housekeeping	2478	Yes	Yes	4%	National Magazines
Homes and Gardens	1324	Yes	Yes	4%	IPC
House and Garden	837	No	Yes	3–4%	Conde Nast
Home and Freezer Digest	1052	Yes	Yes	2%[b]	Beap Ltd
Ideal Home	1673	—	Yes	6%[2]	IPC
The Lady	—	Yes	Yes	Less than 1%	The Lady
Living	1550	—	Yes	8%[b]	International Thomson Ltd
Mother	282	Yes	No	—	IPC
My Weekly	1963	Yes	No	11%[b]	D. C. Thomson
New Health	88[d]	Yes	No	—	Haymarket Publishing

Magazine					Publisher
Parents	478	Yes	No	—	Gemini Publications Ltd
People's Friend	1982	—	Yes	Very rare	D. C. Thomson
Pins and Needles	793	—	Yes	7%[b]	Consumer and Industrial Press
Spare Rib	26[d]	Yes	No	—	Spare Rib Ltd
Woman & Home	2450	Yes	Yes	3%[c]	IPC
Woman's Journal	1050	Yes	Yes	3%[3]	IPC
Woman's Realm	2095	—	Yes	9%	IPC
Woman's Weekly	3275	Yes	No	None	IPC
Woman's Story	409	Yes	Yes	10%	Argus
Working Woman	40[d]	—	Yes	7%[b]	Wintour Publications Ltd

[a]Estimates are from National Readership Survey Jan–June 1984.
[b]Calculated estimate.
[c]IPC unpublished.
[d]Circulation figure, readership figures not available.

readers.' Products in this category include: slimming remedies, breast developers and 'youth enhancers'. *Family Circle* would not allow known hazardous products to be published without attention being drawn to these dangers through, for example, a Government Health Warning.

While not automatically accepting all advertising, Judith Hall, editor of *Woman's Realm* was unique in admitting to accepting advertising for harmful products: 'Yes, I do accept advertising for products known to be hazardous to health: not just for cigarettes but also alcohol—and butter, cream and all dairy products.' Several magazines turned down sex advertisements because they felt they may embarrass their readers. *Vogue* turned down 'revolting' advertisements that are out of keeping with their style as did *Just Seventeen* and *Smash Hits* which would not take advertising for sanitary protection which it claimed 'would be offensive to male readers'. *Homes and Gardens* put its 'unaesthetic' advertisements at the back of the magazine. *Company* refused advertisements which they considered 'deliberately misleading'.

Cigarette Advertising Policy

Thirty-two per cent (17) of the total refused cigarette advertising. The bulk of these (47 per cent) were among the young teenage magazines (Table 1), none of whom accepted cigarette advertising. Tables 2 and 3 show that out of the 23 magazines whose main readership is under 25, only four refused cigarette advertisements, these were *Look Now*, *19*, *Loving* and *Fitness*.

Sixty-four per cent of the magazines accepted cigarette advertising. This accounted for between less than 1 to 14 per cent of the total advertising revenue per issue, an overall average of 7 per cent per issue. Magazines which appeared to have the highest income from cigarettes were *Company* (14 per cent), *Over 21* (13 per cent), *My Weekly* (11 per cent), *Annabel* (10 per cent) and the *Argus Woman's Three** (10 per cent). Nearly all the magazines which accepted cigarette advertising would take all brands. *Vogue* and *Woman's Own* said they would not accept advertisements directly aimed at women, such as *Kim*. *Woman and Home* vetoed campaigns that were 'too dominant',

---

True Story, *Woman's Story*, *True Romances*.

TABLE 5   Magazines with no response from editor

Magazine	Acceptance of cigarette advertising	Approximate revenue from cigarette advertising[a]	Publisher
Annabel	Yes	10%	D. C. Thomson
Honey	Yes	3%	IPC
Fashioncraft	Not known	Not known	Litharne Ltd
Ideal Home	Yes	6%	IPC
Living	Yes	8%	International Thomson Ltd
Mother and Baby	Not known	Not known	D. C. Thomson
Over 21	Yes	13%	M S Publishing
People's Friend	Yes	Very low	D. C. Thomson
Pins and Needles	Yes	7%	Consumer & Industrial Press
Working Woman	Yes	7%	Wintour Publications Ltd

[a]Calculated estimate.

and restricted its advertisements to low-to-middle tar brands. Ten editors did not respond to the letters or telephone messages (Table 5). Eight out of the ten were known to accept cigarette advertisements.

Those magazines which refused cigarette advertising did so mainly on health grounds or because they did not want to encourage young readers to start smoking. It was the stated policy of both D. C. Thomson's and IPC's young teenage magazines (Table 1) that cigarette advertising should not be accepted on the grounds of their young readerships. Phil O'Neil, editor of *No 1*, would not accept cigarette advertising 'because 50 per cent of readers are under the legal smoking age.'* The two specialist health magazines—*Fitness* and *New Health*—were adamant in their refusal of cigarette advertisements on

---

*It is illegal to sell cigarettes to anyone under 16.

health grounds. Melanie Kee of *New Health* regarded it as 'hypocritical' to do so. Isabel Walker, editor of *Fitness*, said: 'We believe that smoking is completely incompatible with fitness. There is no other class of advertising on which we take such a firm stand.' This view was also endorsed by Gerry Fallen, editor of *Loving* who said 'Being very anti-smoking I would never take on any advertising for cigarettes.' David Hepworth, managing director of *Just Seventeen*, took this line further: 'We don't accept advertisements for products known or suspected to be hazardous to health.' IPC's *Woman's Weekly* was the only magazine in the IPC adult women's group that has never accepted cigarette advertising. This was because of a unilateral decision taken by the editor. Laurie Farnham, IPC's Group Sales Manager, explained why IPC felt that *Woman's Weekly* readers should be protected from cigarette advertising: '*Woman's Weekly* readers are homely women, a little older than average, and tend not to venture far into the wide world.'

The reasons which the rest of the magazines gave for accepting cigarette advertising fell into five main categories. First, there were those who saw it as an important source of revenue. Although over 70 per cent did not divulge actual revenue earned, Alison Green, Advertising Manager at IPC with responsibility for *Woman*, emphasized the importance of, if not a total reliance on, the tobacco companies. Bill Williamson, editor of *Ms London* put it simply: 'Although a firm believer in anti-smoking, it isn't always possible to turn down the kind of lucrative advertising the tobacco industry generates.'

Second, many editors felt that it was not their role to act as censors for intelligent readers in what they saw as a free society. Maggie Goodman, editor of *Company* said: 'I assume our readers are informed enough and mature enough to make their own decisions on the subject. In general I do not believe in censoring advertising any more than I believe that editorial should, in any way, be affected by advertising pressure.' This view was reiterated by *Woman's World* and *Woman*. Richard Barber, recently appointed editor of *Woman* said: 'It seems hypocritical to accept cigarette advertisements, but I believe our readership is able to make an adult judgement.' The publisher of *House and Garden*, Glynn Stanford, took the argument even further: 'Conscious of its position within a free society, *House and Garden* has a free and open policy with regard to advertisements.'

Third, some magazines made it clear that if a cigarette advertisement was acceptable to the Advertising Standards Authority (ASA), which pre-vets all cigarette advertisements, then it was acceptable to them. Laurie Purden, editor-in-chief of *Woman's Journal*, believed that cigarette advertisements which reached his magazine could not, in his view, make false claims or be misleading because 'All copy is vetted and accepted or not accepted by the ASA. There are very strict rules governing what can or cannot be said and portrayed in cigarette advertisements.'

Fourth, a few magazines took the view that as long as a cigarette advertisement carried a health warning, then it was acceptable. Jill Churchill, editor of *Family Circle*, said: 'Obviously I would not allow known hazards to be published (through advertising) without attention being drawn to those dangers. Each cigarette advertisement does, of course, carry a Government Health Warning.'

Finally, a minority of editors reluctantly accepted cigarette advertising, but wished that they did not. Charlotte Lessing, editor of *Good Housekeeping*, said: 'I am positively against smoking or any encouragement of it, and wish my company would turn down cigarette advertising.' Deborah Hutton, health editor of *Vogue*, personally would rather see no cigarette advertising at all, but explained that advertising policy was determined by their publishers, Conde Nast: 'I appreciate the contradiction in accepting cigarette advertising. But we do write several articles on smoking and health and cover all the new research.' Iris Burton, editor of *Woman's Own*, did not like accepting cigarette advertising either: 'Personally, I don't like it—my mother died of lung cancer. But we are not in the business of censoring our readers.' They perhaps felt some sympathy with the feeling expressed by editor-in-chief of *True Story* of being 'between the devil and the deep blue sea.' One magazine, *Slimming*, had a unique rationale for accepting cigarette advertising. Its editor, Patience Bulkeley, regarded her magazine as 'scientific', and saw accepting cigarette advertising as a logical consequence of this approach.

Effects of Cigarette Advertising

Although editorial policy on cigarette advertising was often ultimately determined by the editor's personal view, many editors made it clear that their views on the effects of cigarette advertising were equally personal, and not based on scientific evidence. Indeed their views tended to mirror their advertising policy on cigarettes. Those who rejected cigarette advertising—especially the young teenage magazines (Table 1), and health magazines—believed that advertising for cigarettes, like any other product, did its job, and encouraged smoking. *No 1* thought that cigarette advertisements encouraged people to smoke because 'that's what ads are for.' *Fitness* presumed that they were effective or 'otherwise there wouldn't be so many women smokers.' On the other hand, magazines which accepted cigarette advertising tended to either take no view at all, or felt them to be ineffective. *Woman's Story* thought their only function was as an art form. *Woman's World* thought they did not increase smoking overall, but only encouraged brand switching. Laurie Farnham from IPC's advertising department agreed as did *Woman's Own*: 'Although we've done no serious research on this, I don't believe that cigarette advertisements in newspapers and magazines carry any more impact. Television, yes, but magazines, no.'

Several editors from magazines such as *Good Housekeeping* and *Home and Freezer Digest* felt that cigarette advertising was far less glamorous than it used to be, and that it was not directed specifically at women. But Sue Dobson of *Woman and Home* felt that despite the content of cigarette advertisements appearing in women's magazines being the same as those in the rest of the media 'they are directed at women on the basis that they are appearing in the magazine.' *Vogue* pointed out that the magazine itself could act as the image-giver to products advertised in it: 'If an ad is seen in *Vogue* this is as good as a stamp of acceptability.'

One or two magazines—notably *Company*—believed that readers could not exercise a free choice on the issue unless there was complete advertising as well as editorial freedom. *Family Circle* and *Slimming* took this a step further, believing that a ban on cigarette advertising in their magazines might reduce revenue to such an extent that the publication of important articles on readers' health might be curtailed.

Coverage of Smoking and Health

Overall, 37 per cent of magazines had recently produced or planned to produce a major article on smoking and health. Most appeared in general women's magazines. Young teenage magazines gave below average coverage to smoking, and other magazines with the bulk of their readers under 25 gave above average coverage to the subject. Out of eight young teenage magazines only *Jackie* claimed to have recently produced a major article covering smoking and health.[28] Many saw the topic as either irrelevant to youth or not compatible with or appropriate for the style or content of their magazine.

For example, the magazines dedicated to romance (*True Story*, *Woman's Story* and *True Romances*) or pop (*Smash Hits*) did not give space to health articles, and magazines like *Homes and Gardens*, *Ideal Home* and *House and Garden* did not see smoking as an appropriate topic to cover.

Among the general women's interest magazines, *Good Housekeeping*, *Vogue* and *Woman's Own* gave well above average coverage to the subject. Iris Burton of *Woman's Own*, which has had regular features on smoking and health as well as a recent editorial, claimed: 'We give a lot more space to smoking and health than to cigarette advertising.' *Vogue* said: 'We are very sympathetic to the issue and are very committed to its serious coverage.' Les Daley of *Woman's World* was exceptional in the view he took: 'We tend not to cover it as a major issue. We assume our readers know all about the risks, and are intelligent enough to decide whether to smoke or not.'

Editors were adamant that they had complete editorial freedom irrespective of their policy on cigarette advertising. However, of the

TABLE 6   Smoking and health coverage: older teenage and younger women's magazines where the majority of readers were 15–24

Magazine	Acceptance of cigarette advertising	Revenue from cigarette advertising	Smoking and health coverage (recent major articles)	% readers who are daily smokers[a]
Company	Yes	14%[b]	Yes	34
Girl About Town	Yes	Very low	No	—
Honey	Yes	3%	—	30
Look Now	No	None	No	34
19	No	None	Yes	35
Over 21	Yes	13%[b]	—	36
Loving	No	None	Yes	47
Ms London	Yes	Very low	Yes	—

[a]Estimates of daily smoking status are from BMRB, 1984 Target Group Index Vol 26, Tobacco.
[b]Calculated estimate.

seven magazines which derived the highest revenue (10 per cent and above) from cigarettes (*Annabel*, *Company*, *Over 21*, *My Weekly*, *True Romances*, *True Story* and *Woman's Story*) none had given major coverage to smoking the previous year.

Smoking Status and Magazine Readership

Thirty-three per cent of women in the general population (aged 16 and over) are smokers. It can therefore be seen from Tables 6–8 that the teenage and younger readers of *Loving*, *True Romances* and *True Story* had a very high percentage of smokers—bordering on 50 per cent. This is probably a reflection of the social background of the particular readerships of these magazines. For example, the sales manager for *True Story* and *True Romances* explained that their readers tended to be young, working-class women from the North of England. But in every magazine for which data was available, the majority of their readers were non-smokers.

Cigarette Advertising and Smoking Status in Magazines with Predominantly Young Readers

Five out of eight older teenagers' and young women's magazines (all with a majority of readers under 25) accepted cigarette advertising (Table 2). In this group, *Over 21* carried more cigarette advertising than nearly every other magazine in any other category. Table 3 shows that 93 per cent of magazines whose largest readership group was under 25, accepted cigarette advertising. Combining the results from Tables 1–3, an average of 58 per cent of magazines with predominantly young readers accepted cigarette advertising. A comparison of what editors reported to us as the main target age range of their readers compared with actual readership figures (Tables 2 and 3), shows that many considerably underestimated the size of their under 25 readership.

In the light of declared Government, magazine and editorial policies not to expose young people to cigarette advertising, we carried out a further analysis of the proportion of teenagers who read a sample of 14 magazines with young readership profiles (Table 9). Several points emerged. First, half of the magazines in this group

TABLE 7   Smoking and health coverage: young women's magazines where the numerically largest readership group was 15–24

Magazine	Acceptance of cigarette advertisements	Revenue from cigarette advertisements	Smoking and health coverage (recent major articles)	Readers who smoke daily[a] (%)
Annabel	Yes	10%[b]	—	28
Cosmopolitan	Yes	5%	Yes	35
Fitness	No	None	Yes	—
Harpers & Queen	Yes	4%	No	37
Mother & Baby	Not known	Not known	—	—
Options	Yes	'Small' (5%)[b]	No	31
She	Yes	8%	No	26
Slimming	Yes	'Occasionally' (2%)[b]	Yes	33
The Face	Yes	Only 1 ever published	No	—
True Romances	Yes	10%	No	47
True Story	Yes	10%	No	45
Vogue	Yes	3%	Yes	35
Woman	Yes	9%[c]	Yes	36
Woman's Own	Yes	8%[c]	Yes	34
Woman's World	Yes	7%	No	27

[a]Estimates of daily smoking statistics are from BMRB, 1984 Target Group Index Vol 26, Tobacco.
[b]Calculated estimate.
[c]IPC unpublished.

accepted cigarette advertising. In five of these, *Annabel, Over 21, Honey, True Romances* and *True Story*, the proportion of 15–19 year old readers equalled or exceeded those in the 20–40 age group, and in all seven which accepted cigarette advertisements, teenagers formed a substantial proportion of their readers. Despite this evidence, Chris Boyd, Group Advertisement Controller for IPC's Youth Magazine

TABLE 8   Smoking and health coverage—older women's magazines
where the majority of readers were over 25

Magazine	Acceptance of cigarette advertisements	Revenue from cigarette advertisements	Smoking and health coverage (recent major articles)	Readers who smoke daily[c](%)
Family Circle	Yes	4%	No	28
Fashioncraft	—	—	—	—
Good Housekeeping	Yes	4%	Yes	29
Homes and Gardens	Yes	4%	No	32
House and Garden	Yes	3–4%	No	35
Home and Freezer Digest	Yes	2%[a]	Yes	27
Ideal Home	Yes	6%[a]	—	34
The Lady	Yes	Less than 1%	No	—
Living	Yes	8%	—	29
Mother	No	None	Yes	36
My Weekly	Yes	11%[a]	No	33
New Health	No	None	Yes	—
Parents	No	None	Yes	—
People's Friend	Yes	Very low	—	30
Pins and Needles	Yes	7%[a]	—	33
Spare Rib	No	None	Yes	—
Woman & Home	Yes	3%[b]	No	26
Woman's Journal	Yes	3%[b]	Yes	29
Woman's Realm	Yes	9%	Yes	30
Woman's Weekly	No	None	No	28
Woman's Story	Yes	10%	No	—
Working Woman	Yes	7%[a]	No	—

[a]Calculated estimate.
[b]IPC unpublished.
[c]Estimates of daily smoking statistics are from BMRB, 1984 Target Group Index
Vol 26, Tobacco.

Group said: 'There has been a policy with the Young Magazines Group not to carry cigarette advertising. This policy was changed last year with *Honey* magazine only, due to increasing maturity of the readers and a change in editorial direction.'

A breakdown of the smoking rates in 15–19 year old readers (Table 9) produced some interesting and alarming results. Although they must be interpreted with caution due to small sample numbers in several cases, it is hard to avoid the conclusion that readers in this age group had much higher than average smoking rates compared with the general population (30 per cent of all 16–19 year olds smoke).[29] Those magazines whose readers had the highest smoking rates (*Jackie*, *Loving* and *My Guy*) did not accept cigarette advertising, and this may reflect a higher than average working class readership profile. But more alarming still are the high proportions of teenage smokers (over 40 per cent) who read *Company*, *Over 21*, *True Romances* and *True Story*, all of whom accepted cigarette advertising. With the exception of *Company*, Table 9 shows that the 15–19 readership group equalled or was larger than the 20–24 age group in each case. Table 9 also shows that a large proportion of the readers of young teenage magazines are not accounted for in the figures. This is because many readers are under 15, and there is no national information available on the number of under 15s who read magazines.

Extrapolating from the figures in Table 9, 1.2 million 15–19 year old girls are exposed to cigarette advertising in this select group of magazines alone. Moreover, two thirds of those who read magazines with a predominantly youthful profile (Tables 1–3) are non-smokers. And by extrapolation again, at least 1 million female non-smokers aged 15–24 will be exposed to cigarette advertising through this group of magazines.

Images of Smoking in Women's Magazines

It has been suggested that the use of glamorous models smoking cigarettes in editorial pages as well as in films has contributed to the growth of smoking among girls and young women.[30] Although magazines such as *The Face*,[31] and *Company*[32] have recently portrayed glamorous models smoking on their editorial pages, these seem to be more the exception than the rule for both these and other women's magazines. *Cosmopolitan*'s Fashion Editor has said she would never feature cigarettes on her pages because 'it's not good to promote a

TABLE 9   Readership by age and smoking status of 14 teenage and younger women's magazines

Magazine	Female readership[a] (%) 15–19	Female readership[a] (%) 20–24	Target readership age (magazine's view)	Percentage of 15–19 readers who smoke[b]	Percentage all readers who are non-smokers[b]	Acceptance of cigarette advertising
Annabel	15	14	—	25	72	Yes
Blue Jeans	50	10	14–15	—	—	No
Company	18	31	Women in their 20s	42	66	Yes
Cosmopolitan	18	28	—	29	65	Yes
Honey	33	29	—	29	70	Yes
Jackie	44	11	12–15	54	64	No
Look Now	42	39	18–21	29	64	No
Loving	45	19	16–24	100	54	No
My Guy	49	13	13–16	75	67	No
19	53	31	15–30	39	64	No
Over 21	28	30	—	49	70	Yes
Patches	59	15	Young	—	—	No
True Romances	19	18	18–24	50	54	Yes
True Story	15	14	16–34	49	55	Yes

[a]Source: NRS Jan–June/April–September 1984.
[b]source: BARM 1984 Target Group Index. Value Tal…

glamorous image of smoking.'[33] We were, nevertheless, interested in whether magazines, especially youth magazines, had an editorial policy on showing models or personalities smoking. Although we did not specifically ask this question in our survey, several magazines, notably *Jackie*, *Smash Hits* and *Harpers and Queen*, spontaneously reported that it was their policy to avoid portraying fashion models or pop stars smoking cigarettes. Harrison Watson, editor of *Jackie*, said: 'We don't normally show girls smoking in our photo stories, and don't portray it as a common, acceptable habit in our fiction and feature material.'

In a content analysis of the 1984 issues of the two top selling youth magazines, *Smash Hits* and *Just Seventeen*[34] there were few examples of pictures which showed people smoking. Indeed only eighteen photographs out of the several hundred which must have appeared in *Smash Hits* during 1984 showed pop stars smoking or holding cigarettes. Only one picture in *Just Seventeen* showed someone smoking and this was an illustration for a story entitled 'None of my best friends smoke.'

DISCUSSION AND CONCLUSIONS

Our analysis shows that while virtually all magazines operated a screening or vetoing policy on advertising, 64 per cent were prepared to accept cigarette advertising. Many editors profoundly contradicted themselves by rejecting products thought to be hazardous, whilst at the same time, accepting advertisements for cigarettes which are known to cause more premature deaths and ill health than any other single product. Although only a few editors were prepared to acknowledge this paradox, the hostility generated in some cases was evidence enough of editors' awareness and sensitivity to the issue. Editors' concomitant interest in promoting health among readers served only to heighten this contradiction.

Striking too, was many editors' apparent willingness to base their cigarette advertising policies on a personal view of its effects on potential consumers, rather than a careful consideration of the evidence. Those who rejected cigarette advertising not surprisingly believed that it encouraged people to start smoking, and those who accepted cigarette advertising believed it either had no effect or only encouraged people to switch brands. It was not possible, of course, to assess the extent to which editors' views were defences for accepting cigarette advertising rather than genuine beliefs.

The tobacco industry defends tobacco advertising by claiming that cigarette advertising neither increases overall cigarette sales nor creates new smokers, but merely persuades established smokers to switch brands.[35] Yet in a comprehensive review of the evidence, the BMA has argued forcefully that cigarette advertising plays a key role in creating an environment where smoking is seen to be desirable, and that this, along with other social factors acts to encourage people to start smoking, and may defer a decision to stop.[36] The advertising industry itself is less reticent about the aims of cigarette advertising. In a recent editorial on the effectiveness of cigarette advertising, the leading advertising magazine *Campaign* said: 'Everybody whose head is out of the sand knows that advertising is an enormously effective marketing weapon. . . . Everybody agrees that the aim of advertising is not to produce memorable work, but to improve sales, or strengthen the cause of whatever is being advertised.'[37] The tobacco industry itself would be unlikely to spend at least £100 million each year promoting its product, if such methods were ineffective. It should, therefore follow, that any magazine with a real commitment to discourage smoking cannot simultaneously encourage cigarette advertising.

Past research into public attitudes towards smoking confirms this view. While 53 per cent in one study often noticed cigarette advertising in magazines, only 7 per cent noticed anti-smoking advertising as often.[38] This study, commissioned by the Government in 1982 from the Office of Population Censuses and Surveys also showed that the views of editors in our survey lagged considerably behind those of the general public, a majority of whom believed that cigarette advertising increases the social acceptibility of smoking, and favoured a ban on its advertising in magazines.[39] Moreover a Government-commissioned NOP poll in November 1984 showed that the proportion of women favouring a specific ban on cigarette advertising in newspapers and magazines was 57 per cent.[40]

Clearly, the revenue it generates is the most important reason for accepting cigarette advertising. This survey shows that dependence on cigarette advertising is not high. But the total magazine market is dominated by three publishers: IPC, D. C. Thomson and National Magazines, each of whom own numerous titles. IPC, the biggest, earned £4.3 million in cigarette revenue out of a total of £75 million in 1984.[41] Magazines such as *Company* and *Cosmopolitan* (owned by National Magazines) which devoted above average proportions of their pages to advertising earned even more per magazine from tobacco. In 1982 *Cosmopolitan* alone earned its publishers, National Magazines, £300,000 from tobacco advertising.[42]

There are two obvious sources of revenue for magazine publishers: sales and advertising. Because of the decline in sales of many large circulation magazines, it has been argued that revenue from cigarette advertising has become even more precious, and that magazines cannot do without it. Our survey shows this not to be the case, as magazines such as *Woman's Weekly* (IPC) have always prospered without taking cigarette advertising, sales and earnings are soaring for the recently launched *Just Seventeen* and *Smash Hits*.[43,44] Moreover, the recently launched independent magazine *Everywoman* and *Mizz*, IPC's new teenage girl's magazine, both firmly refuse cigarette advertising.[45,46]

A recent industry analysis of the magazine market argues that it is short-sighted to focus only on the steady circulation decline, especially in the women's weeklies, since the 1950s,[47] and that massive circulation magazines are 'the relics of a different past' when prices were artificially held down, other leisure activities restricted, and newsprint rationed: 'It is unrealistic to look back to those (postwar) days especially when the economics of advertising make it more attractive to have a smaller, more carefully targeted magazine for which the consumer and advertiser were prepared to pay substantially more.' It is also widely believed that the loss of revenue resulting from a ban on cigarette advertising would mean the closure of magazines. An analogy has been drawn between the collapse of a number of medical magazines due to recent curbs on drug promotion imposed by the Government.[48] This comparison is invalid because the only real source of advertising revenue for most medical magazines is the drug industry. And for these, unlike the position with women's magazines, there are few realistic alternatives other than raising subscription prices.

Although IPC advertising managers expressed concern to us that a ban on cigarette advertising might mean magazine closures, the evidence suggests that this is unlikely. A survey of the press in 1976 concluded: 'The belief that a ban on cigarette advertising would kill the press is not supported by fact.'[49] It found that not only was 'the inevitability of a ban' accepted, but the press had prepared for it 'by building up revenue from other sources.' Gerry Wynveldt, the then Managing Director of IPC Magazines, said: 'We've got so many magazines that a ban won't really affect us. Tobacco represents a very small proportion of our total advertising revenue, and is declining in some magazines.'[50] In a more recent review both IPC and National Magazines came to the same conclusion and 'consider they have enough revenue from other sources not to worry if cigarette advertising is banned.'[51] Although dependence on cigarette advertising has increased since then magazines today are still unlikely to collapse as a result of a ban on cigarette advertising, because more than 90 per cent of revenue, still comes from non-tobacco sources.

It is also accepted as a truism that the final decision on whether to accept cigarette advertising or not rests with magazine proprietors. Although *Vogue* (Conde Nast) and *Good Housekeeping* (National) claimed this to be the case, all IPC editors insisted that they could veto any form of advertising if they felt strongly enough about it. This is clearly the case with *Woman's Weekly* whose editorial decision not to take cigarette advertising has always been respected by the publishers. Likewise with *Woman and Home* in the 1970s, when its editor decided to refuse cigarette advertising (this decision has since been reversed).

The other reasons given in this survey in support of cigarette advertising are even less defensible. First is the idea, put forcefully by *Company*, that a free society should uphold the right of an advertiser to sell a product, and that readers are somehow unable to make an informed choice about whether or not to smoke without such advertising. This argument could only have currency if there were any controversy about the effects of cigarettes. But the evidence on the dangers of smoking is so overwhelming (and acknowledged to be so by most magazines), and there can be no health argument in favour of smoking. The way to enable readers to make an informed choice about smoking is not through advertising, but through good editorial coverage.

Less defensible still is the argument that there is no reason to reject cigarette advertisements as they have been through a 'rigorous' pre-vetting process by the ASA. First, it is obvious from the survey, that cigarette advertisements constantly slip through the ASA's monitoring system into youth magazines (see below). Second, editors contradict themselves again by rejecting advertisements for other products that they deem have 'slipped' through the ASA's Code of Advertising Practice at the same time as accepting its judgements on cigarettes as the final word. The code's fallibility was clearly demonstrated by the campaign launched in 1982 for *Kim* cigarettes which was deemed by a complainant to breach the ASA's code on cigarettes. The complaint was upheld and the advertisement was withdrawn only to be replaced by a series of similar advertisements which slipped through the code.

Some editors, notably *Family Circle* and *Woman's Journal*, used the presence of a Government Health Warning as a justification for accepting cigarette advertisements. Yet opinion surveys have shown that the presence of a health warning offers little protection against the exhortations of the advertising itself: 97 per cent of women could not even recall the wording of the Health Warning.[52]

Cigarette Advertising Policy and Young Readers

The Government's stated policy is to protect young people from inducement to smoke, and its voluntary agreement with the tobacco industry on tobacco advertising embodies this principle. As part of this voluntary agreement, the ASA has been endowed with the responsibility of monitoring cigarette advertising in print media. The cigarette manufacturers must submit all cigarette advertisements to the ASA first, ostensibly to ensure that they are not in breach of the Code of Advertising Practice for Cigarettes which is part of the ASA's general Code of Advertising Practice.[53] The 'essence' of this code is that 'Advertisements should not seek to encourage people, particularly the young to start smoking. . . . and should not seek to exploit those who are particularly vulnerable, in particular young people.' And rule 2.12 of the code states: 'No advertisement should appear in any publication directed wholly or mainly at young people.'

What is a Young Reader?

Young non-smokers and experimental smokers are the single most important group who should be protected from cigarette advertising. There is little guidance from the Government on what is young, and the ASA code does not define youth although it states in its guidelines for interpreting the code that all models used in cigarette advertising should be over 25. We have therefore adopted the United Nations' designation as 25 for the upper limit of youth. Nearly all those who take up smoking, do so before the age of 25.[54] Most start under the age of 20,[55] but nearly one in five, representing another 140,000 new smokers, start between the ages of 20 and 24.[56]

By this definition, our survey shows that not only the spirit, but the letter of the ASA code is being broken. A total of 63 per cent of magazines with a predominantly under 25 readership profile accepted cigarette advertisements (Tables 2 and 3 combined). This means the tobacco companies have easy access to at least one million non-smokers aged 15–24 through these magazines. A separate analysis of 14 of these magazines (Table 9) revealed that up to 1.2 million 15–19 year old girls are being exposed to cigarette advertisements through this group of magazines alone.

These issues were recently raised with the ASA following two complaints concerning cigarette advertisements appearing in teenage and young women's magazines which were seen to breach Rule 2.12 of the code which precludes advertisements from appearing in 'any publication directed wholly or mainly at young people.' The Council's preliminary conclusion, which took three months of deliberation, was that the United Nations' definition of youth was not 'relevant' to the interpretation of the code, and that 'under 18' was a better working definition, although this is not stated anywhere in the code itself. Furthermore, it decided to postpone any judgement on whether the tobacco companies were in breach of Rule 2.12 because it wanted to study the readership figures more carefully. The ASA code, according to Peter Smith, the ASA's cigarette advertisement assessor, was designed to restrict the content of cigarette advertisements, and not to control the media in which the advertisements appear. Rule 2.12, therefore, 'is the oddball', he said. 'It got dragged into Appendix H (The Cigarette Code), ill-advisedly, in some people's view, and it has stuck since then.'[57] Yet if the 'essence' of the ASA's code is to protect young people from inducements to smoke, our study shows that the ASA is a wholly ineffective vehicle for doing this.

It is clear from our survey that there is no misunderstanding about the youth of the readership of young teenagers' magazines (Table 1), all of which reject cigarette advertising on the grounds that their readers are too young, and therefore vulnerable to cigarette advertising. However, ideas about what is young become confused as the readership age becomes more mixed. IPC's policy on young magazines, supported by both its advertising and editorial departments, is that none of the 'young' magazines should take cigarette advertising. IPC's *Honey*—which started taking cigarette advertisements recently—is no longer a 'young' magazine according to Patricia Lamburn, IPC's editorial director and former Council member of the Health Education Council. Yet it was described in a recent TV programme as 'The first magazine to take teenagers seriously'.[58] Moreover IPC still insists that *Honey*'s readership has become 'older', although 56 per cent of its readers are under 25, most of whom are *under 20*.

In reply to a recent complaint from a doctor about the large number of cigarette advertisements carried by *Over 21*, the editor, Pat Roberts said she was satisfied that no breach of the 'stringent' ASA code had taken place because 'the median age of our readers is 23 years with 90 per cent over the age of 18.'[59] Yet *Over 21*'s problem page is littered with letters from teenagers and 28 per cent of its readers are teenagers.

In a recent effort to direct a Good Health campaign at teenage girls and young women, the Scottish Health Education Group (SHEG) devised a booklet on smoking and health for insertion into young women's magazines. In order to reach a target group of 16–24 the booklets were placed in five magazines with a 'young' readership profile, including two, *Honey* and *Woman's World*, which take cigarette advertising.[60] If these readers are seen by health educators to be young, it is surely unacceptable that they should be treated otherwise by the tobacco industry and magazines.

Reaching Large Numbers of Young Women

Many of the magazines shown in Table 3 (where the numerically largest group of readers were under 25) took the view, like Richard Barber of *Woman*, that their readers were adult enough to make a 'mature' judgement about the merits or otherwise of cigarette advertising. Yet when he was editor of *Look Now*, which had 420,000 readers under 25, he 'wouldn't have dreamed of accepting cigarette advertising. . . . Because at 14 you're more impressionable.' *Woman's Own*, *Cosmopolitan* and *Vogue* each have 600,000–1,000,000 readers under 25. Surely they also have the right to be protected from inducements to smoke. Recent evidence shows that teenhood is no bar to reading adult women's magazines. Two surveys of 12–18 year olds showed that girls start reading women's weeklies and monthlies as early as 13 and 14.[61,62]

The Role of Government

Despite editors' and publishers' real powers of veto over advertising, the ultimate responsibility for controlling the promotional activities of the tobacco industry rests with Government. Several magazines disapproved of cigarette advertising, but would not be prepared to act unilaterally. Jill Churchill of *Family Circle* said: 'Personally I don't like to see cigarette advertising directed at women or anyone else. However, I cannot ban them from our magazine unless, and until, all rival companies publishing magazines agree to ban them too.'

In a recent interview with one of the authors of this study, John Patten MP, Parliamentary Under Secretary of State at the Department of Health, said that he thought the tobacco industry's voluntary agreement with Government was 'largely being observed,' and that the ASA was 'doing a good job' protecting youth from exposure to cigarette advertising 'although there have been problems from time to time, and things slip through the net.'[63] The findings in this survey show that the hole in the ASA's net is as big as a house. Even the ASA itself admitted to us: 'We cannot prevent the actions of advertisers.' This study shows that not only is the tobacco industry riding rough-shod over the voluntary agreement, it is constantly in breach of the 'essence' of the ASA's code which is to protect young non-smokers from cigarette advertising. This not only illustrates the failure of volun-tary agreements to curb the industry's activities, but also that the ASA code itself acts as a bar to effective action aimed at protecting the young from exposure to cigarette advertising. The cigarette manufac-turers, according to Margaret Koumi, editor of 19, which does not take cigarette advertisements, 'take a very moral stand themselves and will not usually use young magazines for their own advertising'. The reality, confirmed by IPC Advertising Staff, is that not only are they gaining access to large numbers of young non-smokers, but magazines with a youthful profile such as Look Now and Honey (which has recently revised its policy and now accepts cigarette advertise-ments), have been under continuing pressure from them to accept cigarette advertising.

The Government's course of action should be clear. The BMA, Royal College of Physicians, World Health Organization, International Union Against Cancer and many other international medical and health bodies have repeatedly called for a ban on all cigarette advertis-ing and promotion. Moreover, experience from Norway and Finland shows that a legislative ban on all tobacco promotion as part of a comprehensive programme had been effective in encouraging big declines in teenage smoking rates and that the sharpest decline of all has been among girls.[64,65]

Smoking and Health Coverage

A survey of health coverage in five major women's magazines throughout 1982 concluded: 'Coverage on smoking and health was strikingly low' with only seven items or articles on smoking out of a total of more than 1000 on health.[66] Things appear to have improved in many ways since then. Our survey shows that more than one third of magazines had recently covered or planned to cover smoking and health, and many gave it news coverage in regular columns. However, this coverage in no way can balance the amount of space given to cigarette advertisements. For example, whilst four items on smoking appeared in the 1984 issues of *Company*, together amounting to one page, approximately 50 pages were given over to cigarette advertisements.[67]

Does the acceptance of cigarette advertising affect editorial freedom to cover smoking and health? Overwhelming evidence from the USA suggests that not only do American magazines which receive large amounts of tobacco revenue play down smoking, but that tobacco companies have brought direct pressure to bear on magazines by withdrawing advertising. A survey of ten major US women's magazines between 1967 and 1979 found only eight major articles on smoking over an entire decade, and four carried none at all over the whole 12 year survey period.[68] A follow-up concluded that the greater the dependence on cigarette advertising, the less likely were they to cover smoking and health.[69] More recently, journalists' coverage of smoking and health in magazines and papers which take cigarette advertising has either been cut down or removed altogether in some instances.[70–72] In one case a journalist was sacked.[73] Tobacco companies appear to have brought direct pressure to bear on *Newsweek* and *Time* magazines—both of whom depend heavily on tobacco revenue. The references to smoking in a personal health supplement in *Newsweek* on November 7th 1983 were de-emphasized because that issue carried $1 million worth of cigarette advertising. Following severe criticisms by medical and health professionals, *Newsweek* published a further health supplement in 1984 which contained a strong statement about the effects of smoking on health. In that issue alone, it lost over half of its usual $1 million tobacco revenue.[74] This experience has been confirmed in Australia where the threat of a legislative ban in tobacco advertising led to editorial compromise in smoking and health coverage.[75]

In Britain there is evidence that the tobacco industry has brought, albeit unsuccessful, pressure to bear on the *Sunday Times* following its coverage of smoking and health in its cigarette advertisement-laden colour supplement. The estimated annual loss of revenue from Imperial Tobacco was £0.5 million.[76] Despite pressure from the tobacco advertisers *Good Housekeeping*'s Editor has ensured that its coverage of smoking remains uncompromised. Two years ago this resulted in a shift of cigarette advertising from an issue which contained an article on smoking to another. In our study editors insisted that they had complete editorial freedom to cover smoking irrespective of their policy on cigarette advertising. But Alison Green, Advertising Manager with special responsibility for *Woman*, said 'The difficulty is that we take money from these people (tobacco companies). It does not matter how much money we take from them, it is difficult for us to endorse anything that goes against the companies. Even editorially, they have to go carefully. The tobacco companies are very sensitive about their image.' This study could not objectively assess whether editorial coverage had ever been compromised by cigarette advertising; some of the most comprehensive coverage of smoking has been in magazines which take cigarette advertising, namely *Cosmopolitan*, *Good Housekeeping*, *Woman's Own* and *Vogue*. But the survey did show that those who derived above average revenue from cigarettes were much less likely to devote any major attention to smoking and health.

It is clear from research[77] that factors other than cigarette advertising influence editorial coverage of smoking. The following have been identified: the style and content of the magazine, the readership profile, personal health experience, contacts with health and medical professionals, and, above all the personal interest of the editor. Our survey confirms many of these observations. While it is possible to appreciate that some specialist magazines on gardening and the home cannot be expected to give smoking much editorial space, it is of considerable concern that only two out of eight young teenagers' magazines give the subject any major coverage.

Some editors, notably Iris Burton of *Woman's Own*, argued that they gave greater editorial space to smoking and health than to cigarette advertising. But for this to be true each IPC weekly would have to devote one to three full editorial pages to the subject in almost every issue! Furthermore, anti-smoking articles which are flanked by cigarette advertising, as they were recently in *Woman's Realm* and *Woman's Own*,[78,79] may strike the reader as if they are not really serious. This is particularly likely to affect smokers, as evidence shows that 44 per cent of smokers believe 'Smoking can't really be dangerous or the Government would ban cigarette advertising.'[80] As the tobacco industry already spends at least 50 times more money promoting smoking than the Health Education Council has to promote non-smoking, it is regrettable that the tobacco companies still have ample opportunity to detract from potentially effective articles on smoking.

REFERENCES

1. Jacobson, B. *The Ladykillers—Why Smoking is a Feminist Issue*. Pluto Press, London 1981.
2. Bewley, B. R. *et al.*, Trends in Children's Smoking. *Community Medicine*, **2**, 186–9, 1980.
3. Rawbone, R. G. *et al.*, Cigarette Smoking Among Secondary School Children, 1975, *Journal of Epidemiology and Community Health*, **32**, 53–58, 1978.
4. Dobbs, J. and Marsh, A. *Smoking Among Secondary School Children*. OPCS, HMSO, London, 1983.
5. Rawbone, R. G. *et al.*, Cigarette Smoking Among Secondary School Children, 1975–79. *Archives of Disease in Childhood*, **57**, 352–58, 1982.
6. Charlton, A. The Brigantia Survey: A General Review. *Public Education About Cancer: Recent Research and Current Programmes 77*, 92–102, 1984.
7. Gillies, P. A. Biosocial Aspects of Smoking in Children and Adolescents. Paper presented to Annual Meeting of British Association for the Advancement of Science, Norwich, Sept. 1984.
8. Ledwith, F. Smoking Prevalence Among Primary and Secondary School Children in Lothian. Proceedings of Health Education and Youth Conference, Southampton, 1982.
9. *General Household Survey 1982*, Office of Population Censuses and Surveys, Social Survey Division, Series GHS No. 12, HMSO, London, 1983.
10. *Ibid.*
11. *The Health Consequences of Smoking for Women, A Report of the Surgeon General*, Washington D.C., US Department of Health, Education and Welfare, 1980.
12. OPCS Mortality Statistics for the UK 1983—partly published.
13. Deaths by Cause. *OPCS Monitor*, June 19, 1984.
14. *Health or Smoking?* Follow-Up Report of the Royal College of Physicians; Pitman Medical Publishing Ltd., London, 1983.
15. Austin, D. Smoking and Cervical Cancer. *Journal of American Medical Association*, **250** (4), 516–17, 22/29 July, 1983.
16. *Health or Smoking? op cit.*
17. *Ibid.*
18. Rogers, D. Editorial, *Tobacco Reporter*, February, 1982.
19. JICNARS, National Readership Survey, 1982.
20. Advertising Association Statistical Yearbook, 1982.
21. Health Education Council, personal communication.
22. White, C. *The Women's Periodical Press in Britain, 1946–1976*. RCOP Working Paper, No. 4, HMSO, 1977.
23. Ferguson, M. *Forever Feminine*. Heinemann, London, 1983.
24. Amos, A. *Matron Advises—Aspects of Health Education in British Women's Magazines*. MSc Thesis, Edinburgh University, Department of Community Medicine, 1983.
25. Amos, A. Women's Magazines and Smoking. *Health Education Journal*, **43**, Nos 2 & 3, 45–50, 1984.
26. Davies, L. and Holdsworth, D. in *Pre-Retirement Education*, Ed. Chris Phillipson, Keele University and Health Education Council, 1983.
27. Amos, A. See ref. 24.

28. Amos, A. Images and Influences in the Media—Positive or negative? Proceedings of a Conference on Smoking in the Late Teens. Hampstead Health Authority, 1985; in press.
29. General Household Survey. *op. cit.*
30. Gillies, P. A. *op. cit.*
31. *The Face*, September and October 1984 and May 1985.
32. *Company*, January, 1984.
33. Wells, I. R. Where There's Smoke. *Blitz*, March 1985.
34. Amos, A. See ref. 28.
35. Waterson, M. J. *Advertising and Cigarette Consumption*. Advertising Association, London, 1984.
36. Chapman, S. *Cigarette Advertising and Smoking: A Review of the Evidence*. B.M.A. Professional Division, March, 1985.
37. How to Stay on a Tightrope. Editorial, *Campaign*, 8 February 1985.
38. Marsh, A. and Matheson, J. *Smoking Attitudes and Behaviour*. An enquiry carried out on behalf of the DHSS, OPCS. Social Survey Division, HMSO, London 1983.
39. *Ibid*.
40. NOP Market Research, 1984, unpublished results from questions commissioned by OPCS.
41. IPC, unpublished.
42. Amos, A. See ref. 25.
43. Teddern, S. Hit and Mizz Theories of Magazine Publishing. *Guardian*, 25th February, 1985.
44. *Campaign*, March 1st 1985.
45. *Everywoman*, personal communication.
46. Health Education Council, personal communication.
47. Bilton, J. Why Today's Magazines are Banking on Visibility. *Campaign*, **17**, 30 September 1983.
48. Hall, D. How the Ill-Wind from Whitehall clobbered the Medical Journals. *Campaign*, March 1, 1985.
49. Ferguson, P. A Cigarette Ban Won't Kill the Press. *Marketing*, 22–25 January 1976.
50. *Ibid*.
51. Cooper, A. Why Women's Magazines are Winning. *Marketing*, 31–37, March 1979.
52. NOP Market Research Ltd, 1981, unpublished results from questions commissioned by OPCS.
53. *The British Code of Advertising Practice*, Appendix H: Advertising of Cigarettes, of the components of manufactured Cigarettes and of Handrolling Tobacco, Advertising Standards Authority, January, 1983.
54. *General Household Survey, op. cit.*
55. Health or Smoking? *op. cit.*
56. Health Education Council, personal communication and General Household Survey, *op. cit.*
57. Advertising Standards Authority, personal communication.
58. 'Will to Win'—A programme about *Working Woman*, Channel 4, January 27, 1985.
59. Dr H. MacAnespie, personal communication.
60. Scottish Health Education Group, personal communication.

61. Davies, E. *Teenage Magazines' Research*. University of London, 1984, unpublished.
62. Balding, J. *Health Related Behaviour Questionnaire*. University of Exeter, personal communication.
63. Jacobson, B. Interview with John Patten M.P. 12/2/85.
64. Lochsen, P. M. *et al.*, *Trends in Tobacco Consumption and Smoking Habits in Norway*. A report from the Norwegian Council on Smoking & Health, Oslo, 1984.
65. Rimpela, M. *Juvenile Health Habits*, University of Helsinki, Finland, in press.
66. Amos, A. See ref. 25.
67. Amos, A. unpublished data.
68. Whelan E. *et al.*, Analysis of Coverage of Tobacco Hazards in Women's Magazines. *Journal of Public Health Policy*, **2**, 28, 1981.
69. Dale, K. C. ACSH Survey: Which Magazines Report The Hazards of Smoking? *ACSH News & Views*, **3**, May/June 1982.
70. Guyan, J. Health Question: Do Publications Avoid Anti-Cigarette Stories to Protect Ad Dollars? *Wall Street Journal*, **22**, November 1, 1982.
71. Transcript '20/20', Growing Up in Smoke, A. Pifer, Producer, ABC Network USA, 20 October, 1983.
72. Whelan, E., *op. cit.*
73. Warner, K. E. Cigarette Advertising and Media Coverage of Smoking and Health. *New England Journal of Medicine*, **312** (6), 384–88, February 7, 1985.
74. *Ibid.*
75. Chapman, S. Cigarette Advertising and Editorial Bias in Australian Newspapers. *Medical Journal of Australia*, **140** (8), 480–82, 1984.
76. Taylor, P. *Smoke Ring—The Politics of Tobacco*. Bodley Head, London, 1983.
77. Amos, A. See ref. 25.
78. Last, P. You Really Can Give Up Smoking. *Woman's Realm*, September, 1984.
79. Rayner, C. What Heavy Smoking Does to Your Body. *Woman's Own*, 16 February, 1985.
80. Marsh, A. and Matheson, J. *op. cit.*

Chapter 4

REPORT ON INVESTMENT IN THE UK TOBACCO INDUSTRY

David Gilbert, Social Audit

Increasing concern about the damaging effects of smoking on health, and growing interest in 'ethical investment', have prompted us to enquire into shareholdings in the UK tobacco industry.

Which are the major companies in the UK industry; and who invests in them? What opportunities might there be for persuading at least some shareholders to invest in more socially useful enterprises?

1. THE UK TOBACCO INDUSTRY

World sales of tobacco products exceed £31 billion/year. British-based companies contribute substantially to this trade.

The UK tobacco industry involves numerous agencies (including, for example, distributors, retailers, advertising and other agencies), but the heart of the industry comprises six major concerns. There are three leading companies, whose connection with tobacco is generally well known:

B.A.T. Industries. Sales of tobacco products accounted for £6138 million—just over half of this company's turnover in 1983. B.A.T. Industries no longer run direct sales and distribution operations in the UK; but they export from Britain, and market over 300 cigarette brands worldwide.

Imperial Group plc accounts for £2420 million sales of tobacco products—i.e. 55 per cent of Group turnover, in 1983. The Imperial Group comprises ten major UK tobacco houses, including John Player and W. D. & H. O. Wills.

Rothmans International and associated companies operate over 40 tobacco factories in Europe and elsewhere. In 1983, £1572 million—nearly 70 per cent of the group's net sales revenue—derived from tobacco.

There are three other companies whose connections with the industry are strong, though probably less well known. These are:

Molins plc, which sells machinery to the tobacco industry. In 1983, the company earned about £100 million from this source, representing 77 per cent of all turnover. As the rest of the company operated at a loss during 1983, the company's tobacco-related business accounted for 173 per cent of profit before tax.

Bunzl plc produces cigarette filters for the domestic and overseas market. The company's Filtrona Division accounted for sales of £90 million—17 per cent of the company's turnover in 1983.

Grand Metropolitan plc owns the US tobacco company, Ligget & Myers. This subsidiary makes a number of 'own brand' and branded cigarettes, including L & M, Chesterfield, Eve and Lark. 'Grand Met' also owns Pinkerton Tobacco Company (chewing and smoking products) and has other tobacco operations in Brazil. Tobacco interests accounted for about £500 million, roughly 10 per cent of all turnover, in 1983.

In January 1984, Grand Metropolitan reported they wanted to sell their interests in tobacco, but a later statement indicates this policy has changed:

'. . . developments in the pricing of cigarettes have prompted Grand Metropolitan USA and the management of the cigarette business to discontinue negotiations' (Company press release dated 20 July 1984).

The Company's annual report for 1983 reported increased tobacco sales in the L & M group for the third consecutive year; and record sales and growth by the Pinkerton and Brazilian subsidiaries.

All six companies are quoted on the London Stock Exchange. Their involvement in tobacco, as summarized above, is communicated to all shareholders in the companies' annual reports.

2. SHAREHOLDINGS IN TOBACCO

The main purpose of our research was to identify shareholders who might respond to appeals not to invest in tobacco companies—bearing in mind the effects of smoking on health.

Though most shareholders in tobacco and other companies are individuals, with holdings usually worth a few hundreds/thousands of pounds, most shares are owned by institutional investors (i.e. insurance companies, pension funds, unit trusts). This report mainly focuses attention on institutional investors—partly because of the size of their investments; and partly for other reasons:

- Institutional shareholders may invest directly on behalf of third parties, many of whom might prefer not to support the promotion of tobacco. For example, employees who contribute part of their earnings to pension funds, are unlikely to include many committed non-smokers.
- Institutional investors may have public responsibilities, which should require them to try to contain rather than encourage use of tobacco. There are obvious reasons, for example, why local authorities might try to avoid investment in tobacco.
- Investment in tobacco may to some extent conflict with the principal stated objectives even of some of the major financial institutions. Fire and life insurance companies are a case in point.

It seems reasonable to assume that both individual and institutional investors are aware at least of concern about the dangers of smoking. Presumably they invest in tobacco in spite of, rather than because of, this. Many shareholders would probably be happy to invest in more socially useful enterprises, provided these offered comparable security and return on investment.

It seems likely therefore that many investors hold shares in tobacco not because they can or would want to defend their position, but because they are not required to defend it. The point is underlined by our finding that many organizations invest in tobacco companies, in spite of clear (and potentially embarrassing) conflict between their investment decisions and their main aims. Investment in the industry by numerous organizations—involved, for example, in health promotion, medical research or child-welfare—gives obvious grounds for concern.

The recent setting up of an 'ethical investment' advisory service, and the UK's first 'ethical investment' unit trust, suggest there are clear alternatives open to those investors—and that the time has come to pursue them.*

---

*The Ethical Investment Research and Information Service (EIRIS, 266 Pentonville Road, London N1 9JY) was set up in 1983. In 1984, Friends' Provident launched the Stewardship Unit Trust (Friends' Provident Unit Life Office, Dorking, Surrey RH4 1QA).

3. RESEARCH METHOD

Company shareholder lists may contain tens of thousands of names, which makes comprehensive searching expensive and impracticable. We therefore developed a list of about 180 'key words' and searched the registers of shareholders only under specific headings—i.e. 'British', 'Royal', 'National' etc.* The list was designed to identify shareholders least likely to be able to justify investment in tobacco.

Many of these investors are identified in this report. They have been listed in the following categories: (1) Health and related areas; (2) Child welfare; (3) Educational establishments; (4) Church and related organizations; (5) General charitable and relief work; (6) Official and national agencies and special interest organizations; (7) Local authorities; (8) Pension funds; (9) Organizations which no longer invest in tobacco.

Some investors were conspicuous by their absence—for example, no major trade union investments were identified. Since beneficiaries can easily invest anonymously, through third parties, this does not necessarily mean that unlisted organizations do not hold shares in tobacco companies. Probably at least one-third of the shares in the major tobacco companies were held on behalf of unnamed beneficiaries, by nominees.

4. INVESTMENTS BY DOCTORS, ETC

Preliminary searches of the registers of shareholders revealed an unexpected number of individual investors identified as 'Dr'. Other titles were found as well. A detailed analysis of a sample of shareholders in the Imperial Group was therefore made.

A 2.22 per cent sample of shareholdings was analysed, and a count made of individuals identified as doctors, members of the clergy or military, titled persons and university professors. As the title 'Dr' may be used by non-medical doctors, the names and addresses of a random sample of 49 shareholders identified as 'Dr' were checked against entries in a medical directory. Of these, about half (24) were identified

---

*Shareholders in the Imperial Group were not listed in the traditional alphabetical order, therefore a modified 'key word' search had to be used. To compensate, two special searches (for county councils and doctors) were carried out on the Imperial File.

as practising medical doctors, and a further 8 were medical doctors who had retired. The remaining one third of the sample (17/49) could not be identified as physicians.

The following estimates were made of the numbers of individuals in each category holding shares in the Imperial Group:

1622 officers in the armed services
1171 practising (856) and retired (315) medical doctors
 721 titled persons (i.e. 'Sir', 'Lord', 'Dame')
 405 members of the clergy
 225 university professors

In addition, an estimated 270 practising and retired doctors sold shares in the Imperial Group in 1983/4.

5. ANALYSIS OF DIVESTMENT

Is there any evidence that investors have sold shares in tobacco, specifically in response to publicity relating to smoking and health?

The analysis of individual shareholdings (above) was based only on existing shareholdings. However, analysis of shares sold in the most recent accounting period (1983/4) did not suggest that doctors were more likely to sell shares in tobacco companies than were other investors:

Analysis of divestment

Class of Investor	Percentage of sample selling tobacco shares in 1983/4
Doctors	19
Clergy	18
Military	14
Titled/professorial	00

A more detailed analysis of share sale dates in five of the six companies was made.* There was no clear evidence of selling concen-

*The register of shareholders in B.A.T. Industries recorded who had sold shares, but not the date of sale.

trated at any particular time of the year. Adverse publicity probably affects levels of investment and divestment in tobacco throughout the year. But there is little evidence to suggest that shareholders would promptly sell their stock in response to new publicity about the ill-effects of smoking on health. During 1983/4, share sales were recorded at the following times of year.

Percentage of share sales by month (1983/4)

JAN	FEB	MAR	APR	MAY	JUN	JUL	AUG	SEP	OCT	NOV	DEC
20	7	7	12	10	0	10	10	7	5	7	5

The analyses of shareholders in the lists that follow are based on searches made in Companies House (Cardiff and London) in September 1984. Share transactions may have taken place since then: enquiries about this should be directed to the organizations concerned.

The symbol [*] in the lists indicates that an entry appears in more than one category. The key indicating size of shareholding is as follows:

Nil	=	Shares no longer held (previous holding)
00	=	Up to 100 shares held
000	=	Up to one thousand shares held
0000	=	One or more thousands of shares held
00000	=	One or more tens of thousands of shares held
000000	=	One or more hundreds of thousands of shares held
0000000	=	One to ten million shares held
00000000	=	Over ten million shares held

6. EXAMPLES OF INSTITUTIONS/AGENCIES INVOLVED IN HEALTH AND RELATED AREAS RECORDED AS HOLDING SHARES IN THE TOBACCO INDUSTRY, AT SEPTEMBER 1984

A number of hospitals, area health authorities, medical schools, professional medical associations and also two major cancer charities were identified among other organizations with health interests owning shares in tobacco. The relatively high level of investment in Grand Metropolitan may be due to the fact that this company's business in tobacco is generally less well known.

Investor	Investment in	Size of Holding
British Dental Association Trust Fund	Grand Met.	0000
British Heart Foundation	Grand Met.	00000
British Home and Hospital for Incurables	Imperial Group	00000
British Kidney Patient Association Investment Trust	Imperial Group	00000
Central Manchester Health Authority	Grand Met.	0000
Charing Cross Hospital Medical School[*]	Grand Met.	0000
Chartered Society of Physiotherapy	Imperial Group	0000
Cheadle Royal Hospital Nominees	Imperial Group	00000
The Governors of Christ's Hospital	B.A.T. Industries	00000
	Grand Met	00000
	Imperial Group	00000
Christadelphian Home and Hospital	Grand Met.	0000
Companions of Britain's Rheumatic and Arthritic Sufferers	Grand Met.	000
Durham Health Authority	Grand Met.	000
Greenwich Health Authority	B.A.T. Industries	0000
	Imperial Group	0000

Investor	Investment in	Size of Holding
Greater Yarmouth & Waveney Health Authority	Grand Met.	000
Greater Glasgow Health Board	Grand Met.	00000
Humberside Contributory Health Scheme	Imperial Group	00000
Imperial Cancer Research Fund	Grand Met.	000000
The Infantile Paralysis Fellowship	Grand Met.	0000
Institute of Cancer Research (Royal Cancer Hospital, SW7)	Grand Met.	00000
King Edward VII Hospital for Officers, London W1	Imperial Group	0000
King's College London School of Medicine and Dentistry[*]	Grand Met.	00000
Liverpool Bluecoat Hospital	Grand Met.	0000
London Hospital Medical College[*]	Grand Met.	0000
The Medical and Dental Defence of Scotland Ltd	Grand Met. Imperial Group	0000 00000
The Medical and Dental Defence Union Ltd (London)	Grand Met.	00000
Medical Protection Society Ltd	Grand Met.	00000
The Medical Research Council[*]	Grand Met.	00000
Merton & Sutton Health Authority	Imperial Group	0000
National Association for Mental Health	Imperial Group	00000
Norwich Health Authority	Imperial Group	0000
Provincial Hospital Services Association (Bedford)	Grand Met.	0000
Queen Charlotte's Hospital for Women	Grand Met.	0000
Royal College of Nursing of UK	Grand Met.	0000
Royal College of Pathologists	Grand Met.	0000
Royal College of Psychiatrists	Grand Met.	0000

Investor	Investment in	Size of Holding
Royal College of Surgeons of Edinburgh	Imperial Group	00000
Royal College of Veterinary Surgeons	Grand Met.	00000
Royal Medical Benevolent Fund	Grand Met.	00000
Royal National Pension Fund for for Nurses[*]	B.A.T. Industries	000000
	Grand Met.	000000
	Imperial Group	000000
Royal Postgraduate Medical School Hammersmith Hospital[*]	Imperial Group	00000
Royal Society for Home Relief to Incurables (Edinburgh)	Grand Met.	0000
	Imperial Group	0000
Royal Surgical Aid Society	Imperial Group	00000
Rugby Health Authority	B.A.T. Industries	0000
The Secretary of State for Defence, Greenwich Hospital[*]	B.A.T. Industries	000000
	Grand Met.	000000
	Imperial Group	00000
Southern Derbyshire Health Authority	Imperial Group	000
South Tees Health Authority	Imperial Group	0000
South West Hertfordshire Health Authority	Imperial Group	0000
Tunbridge Wells Health Authority	Molins	0000
Welsh National School of Medicine	Grand Met.	0000
West Dorset Health Authority	Imperial Group	0000
Westfield Contributory Health Scheme	Imperial Group	00000

7. ORGANIZATIONS AND INSTITUTIONS CONCERNED WITH CHILDREN'S WELFARE RECORDED AS HOLDING SHARES IN THE TOBACCO INDUSTRY, AT SEPTEMBER 1984

It is generally accepted that children should be encouraged *not* to start smoking—and there is corresponding concern about promotion for tobacco products which may encourage the habit among young people. Public policy in this area is underlined by law which prohibits the sale of tobacco to children aged under 16 years old. There seems to be little if any justification for investment in tobacco by any organization concerned primarily with childrens' welfare.

Investor	Investment in	Size of Holding
The Catholic Children's Society[*]	B.A.T. Industries	0000
Catholic Child Welfare Society (Headingley, Leeds, Hallam)[*]	B.A.T. Industries	0000
	Grand Met.	0000
	Imperial Group	0000
Children's Country Holiday Fund	Imperial Group	00000
The Churches and Universities (Scotland) Widows and Orphans Fund[*]	Bunzl	00000
The Church of England Children's Society[*]	Grant Met.	00000
	Imperial Group	00000
The Fellowship of St Nicholas Homes For Children	Imperial Group	0000
Girls' Venture Corps (Surrey)	Grant Met.	0000
Governors of the Dean Orphanage and Calvin's Trust, Edinburgh	Imperial Group	0000
Infantile Paralysis Fellowship[*]	Grand Met.	0000
The Insurance Orphan Funds	B.A.T. Industries	00000
	Grand Met.	00000
	Imperial Group	00000

Investor	Investment in	Size of Holding
National Society for the Prevention of Cruelty to Children	Imperial Group	00000
National Star Centre for Disabled Youth Ltd., Cheltenham[*]	B.A.T. Industries	000
North East Children's Society	Imperial Group	0000
The Royal Liverpool Seamen's Orphans Institution	Grant Met. Imperial Group	00000 00000
The Royal Masonic Institution for Boys	B.A.T. Industries	00000
The Royal Masonic Institution for Girls	Rothmans B.A.T. Industries Imperial Group	00000 000000 00000
The Royal School for Deaf Children	Grand Met. Imperial Group	0000 0000
Royal Soldiers' Daughters Home	B.A.T. Industries Imperial Group	0000 0000
Sailors' Orphans Society of Scotland	B.A.T. Industries	0000

8. EXAMPLES OF EDUCATIONAL ETC. ESTABLISHMENTS RECORDED AS HOLDING SHARES IN THE TOBACCO INDUSTRY, AT SEPTEMBER 1984

For essentially the same reasons as stated in section 7 above, investment in tobacco companies by educational establishments appears illogical and unjustifiable. Conflict of interest is underlined by the use of disciplinary and other measures in schools, aimed at stopping students from smoking. The case for responsible shareholding by universities in the US has been discussed at length elsewhere (Simon, J. G., Powers, C. W. and Gunneman, J. P., *The Ethical Investor, Universities and Corporate Responsibility* (New Haven, Conn.: Yale University Press, 1972).

Investor	Investment in	Size of Holding
Chancellor, Masters and Scholars of the University of Oxford	Imperial Group	000000
Charing Cross Hospital Medical School[*]	Grand Met.	0000
College of St Barnabus (Lingfield, Surrey)	Imperial Group	00000
Incorporated Association of Preparatory Schools Aberfan Trust	Imperial Group	0000
Incorporated Guild of Cheltenham Ladies College	Grand Met.	000
Church Schoolmasters and School-Mistresses Benevolent Institution	Imperial Group	000
Clifton College, Bristol	Imperial Group	0000
Dulwich College Mission[*]	Grand Met. Imperial Group	000 0000
Eastbourne College	Imperial Group	0000
Friends of Highgate School Society	Grand Met.	0000
Girls' Educational Co Ltd (Wycombe Abbey School)	Grand Met.	00000
The Governing Body of Rugby School	Imperial Group	00000
The Governing Body of Shrewsbury School	Imperial Group	0000
Governors of the Dumfrieshire Educational Trust	B.A.T. Industries	0000
Haileybury and Imperial Service College (Hertford)	Grand Met.	0000
Imperial College of Science and Technology	B.A.T. Industries	0000
King's College London School of Medicine and Dentistry[*]	Grand Met.	00000
King Edward VI School (Birmingham)	Grand Met.	00000
London Business School Trust Co.	Imperial Group	00000

Investor	Investment in	Size of Holding
London Diocesan Board for Schools[*]	Imperial Group	0000
London Hospital Medical College[*]	Grand Met.	0000
London House for Overseas Graduates	Grand Met.	00000
London School of Economics	B.A.T. Industries	00000
	Grand Met.	00000
Manchester College, Oxford	Grand Met.	0000
The Masters, Fellows and Scholars in the University of Cambridge	Grand Met.	00000
The President and Fellows of New Hall, University of Cambridge	Grand Met.	0000
The President and Fellows of Queen's College, Cambridge	Grand Met.	0000
Principal and Fellows of St Hilda's, Oxford	Grand Met.	0000
The Principals, Tutors and Professors of St David's College, Lampeter	Imperial Group	0000
The Provost, Fellows & Scholars of Worcester College, Oxford	B.A.T. Industries	0000
The Provost and Scholars of Oriel College, Oxford	Rothmans	0000
	Imperial Group	0000
Queen's University of Belfast	B.A.T. Industries	00000
	Grand Met.	00000
	Imperial Group	00000
The Rector and Fellows of Lincoln College, Oxford	Imperial Group	00000
Royal Alexander and Albert School (Reigate, Surrey)	Grand Met.	0000
Royal Agricultural College (Cirencester, Glos.)	Grand Met.	00000
	Imperial Group	000
The Royal Blind & Asylum School	Bunzl	00000
Royal Holloway College, University of London	Grand Met.	0000

Investor	Investment in	Size of Holding
Royal Postgraduate Medical School Hammersmith Hospital[*]	Imperial Group	00000
The Royal Wanstead School	Rothmans	00000
Rugby School	Grand Met.	0000
School of Oriental and African Studies	B.A.T. Industries	0000
St Catherine's College, University of Oxford	Imperial Group	0000
St David's, University College of Lampeter	Imperial Group	0000
Shrewsbury School	Grand Met.	0000
Truro Cathedral School	Imperial Group	000
University College, Cardiff	B.A.T. Industries	0000
University College of Southampton	B.A.T. Industries	00000
The University College of Wales	Rothmans	00000
	B.A.T. Industries	00000
University of Aberdeen	Imperial Group	00000
University of Bristol	Grand Met.	00000
University of Durham	Bunzl	00000
University of Exeter	Imperial Group	0000
University of Glasgow	Imperial Group	000000
	Grand Met.	00000
University of Hull	Imperial Group	00000
	Grand Met.	00000
University of Leeds	Imperial Group	00000
	Grand Met.	00000
University of Leicester	Imperial Group	
University of London	Bunzl	00000
University of Nottingham	Imperial Group	00000
	Grand Met.	00000
University of Reading	Grand Met.	00000
University of Southampton	Grand Met.	00000
University of Wales	Grand Met.	0000

Investor	Investment in	Size of Holding
Victoria University of Manchester	Grand Met.	000000
Victoria University of Manchester	Grand Met.	000000
	Imperial Group	000000
Westfield College, University of London	Imperial Group	0000

9. EXAMPLES OF CHURCH AND RELATED ORGANIZATIONS RECORDED AS HOLDING SHARES IN THE TOBACCO INDUSTRY, AT SEPTEMBER 1984

The churches have an important and long-standing interest in healing and the relief of suffering. Investment in businesses which promote dangerously unhealthy practices does not benefit the community, and may diminish the credibility and moral authority of church and related organizations.

Investor	Investment in	Size of Holding
Additional Curates Society	Molins	00000
Anglo-Jewish Association	Grand Met.	00
Birmingham Roman Catholic Diocesan Trustees	Imperial Group	0000
The Bishop of Norwich	Grand Met.	00000
	Imperial Group	00000
Blackburn Diocesan Board of Finance	Imperial Group	0000
Board of Guardians for the Relief of the Jewish Poor[*]	B.A.T. Industries	0000
Bristol Diocesan Board of Finance Ltd	B.A.T. Industries	0000
	Imperial Group	0000

Investor	Investment in	Size of Holding
The Catholic Children's Society[*]	B.A.T. Industries	0000
Catholic Child Welfare Society (Headingley, Leeds, Hallam)[*]	B.A.T. Industries	0000
	Grand Met.	0000
	Imperial Group	0000
Central Board of Finance of the Church of England	Imperial Group	0000
Chapter of the Order of the Holy Paraclete (St Hilda's Priory)	Imperial Group	0000
Chelmsford Diocesan Board & Board of Finance	Imperial Group	0000
Cheshire Congregational Union	Imperial Group	0000
Chichester Diocesan Board	Imperial Group	0000
The Church Army	Grand Met.	0000
	Imperial Group	000
The Churches and Universities (Scotland) Widows and Orphans Fund[*]	Bunzl	00000
Church Moral Aid Association	B.A.T. Industries	0000
The Church of England Children's Society[*]	Grand Met.	00000
	Imperial Group	00000
Church Schoolmasters and Schoolmistresses Benevolent Institution	Grand Met.	000
	Imperial Group	000
Clifton Catholic Diocesan Trustees	Imperial Group	00000
Congregational Union of England and Wales	Grand Met.	0000
Congregational Union of Scotland	Imperial Group	0000
The Dean and Chapter of the Cathedral Churches of:		
Chester	Imperial Group	0000
Christchurch, Oxford	Imperial Group	00000
Ely	Imperial Group	0000
Exeter	Imperial Group	0000
St Peter, Exeter	Imperial Group	0000

Investor	Investment in	Size of Holding
Litchfield	Imperial Group	0000
Liverpool	Imperial Group	00000
Devon & Cornwall Congregational	Imperial Group	0000
Dulwich College Mission[*]	Grand Met.	000
Friends of the Clergy Corporation	B.A.T. Industries	000000
	Imperial Group	00000
Gloucester Diocesan Association for the Deaf	Imperial Group	000
Gloucester Diocesan Trust Ltd	Imperial Group	000
Guildford Diocesan Board of Finance	B.A.T. Industries	000
The London Baptist Property Board	Imperial Group	0000
The London Diocesan Board for Schools	Imperial Group	0000
London Diocesan Fund	Grand Met.	000
	Imperial Group	0000
The Lord Bishop of Derby	Grand Met.	000
Manchester Diocesan Board of Finance	Imperial Group	0000
Manchester District Association of Unitarian and Free Christian Churches	Imperial Group	0000
The Methodist Chapel Aid Association Ltd (York)	Grand Met.	0000
Methodist Missionary Trust Association	B.A.T. Industries	00000
National Council of YMCAs Inc.	Grand Met.	0000
	Imperial Group	0000
Nottingham Roman Catholic Diocesan Trustees	Imperial Group	0000
Portsmouth Diocesan Board of Finance	Imperial Group	0000
The Rector and Churchwardens of:		
Combe Florey Parish Church	Imperial Group	000

Investor	Investment in	Size of Holding
The Parish of Birdbrook	Imperial Group	0000
The Parish of Haslemere	Imperial Group	0000
St Mary's the Virgin, Ashford, Kent	Imperial Group	000
Representative Church Body	Rothmans	000
Church of Ireland	Imperial Group	00000
Representative Body of the Church in Wales	Imperial Group	0000
Representative Church Council of the Episcopal Church in Scotland Trustees' Nominees	B.A.T. Industries	0000
Rochester & Southwark Diocesan Board	Imperial Group	0000
Scottish Episcopal Church Nominees	Grand Met.	00000
Secular Clergy Common Fund Ltd	B.A.T. Industries	00000
Sheffield Diocesan Board of Finance	Imperial Group	0000
Sisters of Charity (Milltown Dublin)	Imperial Group	00000
Sisters of Mercy, Sheffield Trustees	B.A.T. Industries	00000
	Grand Met.	00000
Society for the Promotion of	Imperial Group	00000
Christian Knowledge	Grand Met.	0000
The Society of the Inner Light	Imperial Group	0000
Society of the Salutation of Mary the Virgin	Imperial Group	0000
Southwark Roman Catholic Diocesan Corporation	Imperial Group	00000
Student Christian Movement of Great Britain and Ireland	Imperial Group	000
Surrey Congregational Union	Imperial Group	000
Truro Diocesan Board of Finance	Imperial Group	0000
Trustees for the Congregation of Religions of the Assumption	Grand Met.	0000
Trustees of the Sacred Heart Sisters	Molins	00000

Investor	Investment in	Size of Holding
Trustees for Methodist Church Purposes, Manchester	B.A.T. Industries	0000
	Imperial Group	0000
	Grand Met.	000
Trustees for Roman Catholic Church Purposes	Imperial Group	0000
	Grand Met.	00000
Trustees for the Franciscan Missionaries of Mary	Imperial Group	0000
Trustees for the Missionaries of St Francis de Sales	Imperial Group	000
Trustees of the Canons Regular of the Lateran	Imperial Group	000
Trustees of the Presbyterian Church in Ireland	Imperial Group	0000
Trustees of the Sacred Heart Sisters (Woodford Bridge, Essex)	B.A.T. Industries	00000
	Imperial Group	00000
	Grand Met.	00000
Trustees of the West London Synagogue of British Jews	Grand Met.	00
United Society for the Propagation of the Gospel	Grand Met.	00000
United Synagogues Trust Ltd	B.A.T. Industries	00000
Wesleyan and General Trustees Ltd	Imperial Group	000000

10. EXAMPLES OF INSTITUTIONS/AGENCIES INVOLVED IN GENERAL WELFARE/RELIEF WORK RECORDED AS HOLDING SHARES IN THE TOBACCO INDUSTRY, AT SEPTEMBER 1984

There may be no direct conflict between the main aims of these organizations and investment in tobacco, but neither could such shareholdings readily be justified as furthering the investor's main aims. Many of the organizations listed below ask for and receive contributions from the general public: probably many donors would not want their contributions invested in tobacco.

Investor	Investment in	Size of Holding
Birmingham Voluntary Service Council	Imperial Group	0000
Board of Guardians for the Relief of the Jewish Poor[*]	B.A.T. Industries	0000
Bristol Royal Society for the Blind	B.A.T. Industries	0000
	Imperial Group	0000
British Paraplegic Sports Society	Grand Met.	0000
	Imperial Group	000
Cheltenham Old People's Housing Society	Imperial Group	00000
City of Bristol Guild of the Handicapped	Imperial Group	0000
Cobtree Charity Trust	Imperial Group	00000
Ex-Services Mental Welfare Society	B.A.T. Industries	0000
Family Welfare Association	B.A.T. Industries	00000
Glasgow Society for Education of the Deaf	Imperial Group	0000
Greater London Fund for the Blind Trustee Co. Ltd	Grand Met.	000

Investor	Investment in	Size of Holding
Incorporated Homes for Ladies with Limited Income	Grand Met.	0000
Ipswich Blind Society	Imperial Group	0000
League of Welldoers	Imperial Group	00000
Liverpool Council of Social Service	Imperial Group	000000
Metropolitan Society for the Blind	B.A.T. Industries Grand Met.	0000 0000
National Council for the Blind of Ireland	Imperial Group	0000
National Benevolent Institution	Grand Met.	00000
National Council for Voluntary Organisations	Grand Met.	00000
National Star Centre for Disabled Youth Ltd, Cheltenham[*]	B.A.T. Industries	000
Naval Benevolent Trust	B.A.T. Industries	00000
Northampton Town and County Blind Association	Grand Met.	0000
Officers' Family Fund	Grand Met.	0000
The Official Custodian for Charities[*]	B.A.T. Industries Rothmans Molins Grand Met.	00000 000000 00000 0000000
People's Dispensary for Sick Animals	B.A.T. Industries Grand Met.	00000 00000
RAF Benevolent Fund	B.A.T. Industries	0000
Royal Agricultural Benevolent Institution, Oxford	Grand Met.	00000
Royal Artillery Charitable Fund	B.A.T. Industries Imperial Group	00000 00000
Royal Commonwealth Society for the Blind	Grand Met.	0000
Royal London Society for the Blind	Grand Met. Imperial Group	0000 00000

Investor	Investment in	Size of Holding
Royal National Lifeboat Institution	B.A.T. Industries	00000
	Bunzl	00000
	Rothmans	00000
	Grand Met.	00000
	Imperial Group	0000
Royal Naval Benevolent Institution, London	Grand Met.	0000
Royal Naval Benevolent Institution, Brompton	Grand Met.	00000
Royal Society for the Prevention of Cruelty to Animals	B.A.T. Industries	0000
	Grand Met.	00000
	Imperial Group	0000
Royal Society for the Relief of Indigent Gentlewomen of Scotland	Imperial Group	00000
St Dunstan's	Imperial Group	0000
The Samaritans	B.A.T. Industries	000

11. EXAMPLES OF OFFICIAL AND NATIONAL AGENCIES AND SPECIAL INTEREST ORGANIZATIONS RECORDED AS HOLDING SHARES IN THE TOBACCO INDUSTRY, AT SEPTEMBER 1984

None of the organizations listed below appears to have any good reason for investment in the tobacco industry; and some have good reason to avoid it. As representative or membership organizations, many of these agencies invest on behalf of people who would prefer not to profit from successful promotion of tobacco.

Investor	Investment in	Size of Holding
Bank of England Nominees	Bunzl	00000
The Biochemical Society	Grand Met.	00000
British Benefit Society	B.A.T. Industries	00000
British College of Ophthalmic Opticians	Grand Met.	0000
The British Ecological Society	Rothmans	0000
The British & Foreign Unitarian Association Inc	Grand Met.	0000
City of Glasgow Friendly Society Trustee Ltd	B.A.T. Industries	00000
The Cremation Society of Great Britain Ltd	B.A.T. Industries	0000
Department of Finance and Personnel, Northern Ireland	Bunzl	0000
Eugenics Society	B.A.T. Industries	0000
Imperial War Graves Endowment Fund Trustees	Bunzl Grand Met.	0000 00000
Institute for Personal Development	Grand Met.	00
Institute of Marine Engineers Guild of Benevolents	Grand Met.	0000
Institution of Fire Engineers	Imperial Group	000
Institute of Journalists	Imperial Group	0000
Institute of Physics	Imperial Group	0000
Institute of Mechanical Engineers	Rothmans Imperial Group	00000 00000
Labour Party Nominees Ltd	Grand Met.	00000
The London Library	B.A.T. Industries Imperial Group	00000 00000
The Medical Research Council[*]	Grand Met.	00000
Minister of Agriculture, Fisheries and Food	B.A.T. Industries	00000
National Library of Wales	Imperial Group	0000

Investor	Investment in	Size of Holding
National Secular Society	Imperial Group	0000
National Society for Abolition of Cruel Sports Ltd	Grand Met.	00000
The Official Custodian for Charities[*]	B.A.T. Industries	00000
	Grand Met.	0000000
	Rothmans	000000
	Molins	00000
The Official Solicitor to the Supreme Court	Grand Met.	0000
The Public Trustees	Rothmans	0000
	Grand Met.	0000
Royal Anthropological Institution of Great Britain and Ireland	Imperial Group	0000
Royal Entomological Society of London	Imperial Group	000
Royal Historical Society	B.A.T. Industries	0000
Royal Humane Society	B.A.T. Industries	0000
Royal Scottish Society for the Arts	Imperial Group	0000
Royal Society for Nature Conservation	Imperial Group	0000
Royal Society of London	B.A.T. Industries	00000
	Imperial Group	0000
Royal Society of Musicians	B.A.T. Industries	0000
Royal Yachting Association	B.A.T. Industries	0000
The Secretary of State for Defence, Greenwich Hospital[*]	B.A.T. Industries	000000
	Grand Met.	00000
The Secretary of State for Education and Science	Grand Met.	0000
The Yorkshire Naturalists Trust Ltd	Rothmans	0000
The Working Ladies Guild	B.A.T. Industries	0000

12. EXAMPLES OF LOCAL AUTHORITIES RECORDED AS HOLDING SHARES IN THE TOBACCO INDUSTRY, AT SEPTEMBER 1984

The majority of local authorities invest in tobacco companies: for example, 37 of 65 UK county and regional councils (57 per cent) held shares in the Imperial Group alone. Other authorities are thought to invest anonymously, through nominees. Investments of £ tens of millions are involved.

The funds invested by local authorities are mainly employee benefits (wages deferred as pensions), and are paid for through the rates. Councils therefore invest on behalf of the community—including probably many who would prefer funds to be invested elsewhere. Local authority investment in the tobacco industry appears to conflict with a number of statutory and other responsibilities—relating for example to public health and safety; education and general community welfare; and environmental health, sanitation and cleansing.

Investor	Investment in	Size of Holding
Avon County Council	Imperial Group	00000000
Berkshire County Council	B.A.T. Industries	00000000
	Imperial Group	0000000
Cambridgeshire County Council	Imperial Group	000000
Central Regional Council, Stirling	Rothmans	000000
	B.A.T. Industries	000000
	Imperial Group	000000
City of Bristol	Imperial Group	00000
City of Edinburgh District Council	B.A.T. Industries	00000
City of Glasgow District Council	Imperial Group	00000
City of London	Grand Met.	000000
City of London	Grand Met.	000000
	Imperial Group	000000

Investor	Investment in	Size of Holding
Clywd County Council	B.A.T. Industries	00000
	Rothmans	00000
	Imperial Group	000000
Cornwall County Council	Molins	000000
Cumbria County Council	Imperial Group	000000
Derbyshire County Council	B.A.T. Industries	000000
	Grand Met.	000000
Devon County Council	Imperial Group	000000
Dorset County Council	B.A.T. Industries	0000000
	Imperial Group	000000
Dyfed County Council	B.A.T. Industries	000000
	Imperial Group	000000
Dundee District Council	Grand Met.	0000
Durham County Council	Grand Met.	000000
	Imperial Group	000000
East Sussex County Council	Imperial Group	000000
Edinburgh District Council	Grand Met.	00000
Fife Regional Council	Imperial Group	000000
Gloucestershire County Council	Imperial Group	000000
Grampian Regional Council	Imperial Group	000000
Greater London Council	Bunzl	000000
	Grand Met.	0000000
Gwent County Council	Rothmans	000000
	Imperial Group	000000
Gwyned County Council	Rothmans	000000
	Imperial Group	000000
Hereford & Worcester County Council	Grand Met.	000000
	Imperial Group	000000
Humberside County Council	Imperial Group	000000
Kent County Council	Imperial Group	000000
Leicestershire County Council	Imperial Group	000000
Local Authorities Mutual Investment Trust	Grand Met.	000000

Investor	Investment in	Size of Holding
London Boroughs of:		
Barking and Dagenham	B.A.T. Industries	000000
	Grand Met.	00000
	Imperial Group	00000
Barnet	Grand Met.	000000
Brent	Grand Met.	000000
Bromley	B.A.T. Industries	000000
	Grand Met.	000000
Camden	Grand Met.	000000
City of Westminster	Grand Met.	000000
	B.A.T. Industries	000000
	Imperial Group	000000
Croydon	Grand Met.	000000
	Imperial Group	000000
Enfield	B.A.T. Industries	000000
	Grand Met.	000000
	Imperial Group	000000
Greenwich	Imperial Group	00000
Hammersmith & Fulham	B.A.T. Industries	000000
	Grand Met.	000000
	Imperial Group	000000
Harrow	Grand Met.	000000
Hounslow	B.A.T. Industries	000000
	Grand Met.	000000
Lambeth	Grand Met.	000000
Lewisham	Grand Met.	000000
	Imperial Group	000000
Merton	B.A.T. Industries	000000
	Grand Met.	00000
	Imperial Group	000000
Newham	Grand Met.	000000
	Imperial Group	000000
Redbridge	Grand Met.	000000

Investor	Investment in	Size of Holding
Tower Hamlets	Grand Met.	00000
	Imperial Group	000000
The Lord Mayor and Citizens of the City of Portsmouth	B.A.T. Industries	0000
Lothian Regional Council	Imperial Group	000000
Merseyside County Council	Imperial Group	0000
Mid-Glamorgan County Council	Imperial Group	000000
Northumberland County Council	Grand Met.	000000
	Imperial Group	000000
Powys County Council	Imperial Group	000000
Shropshire County Council	B.A.T. Industries	000000
	Grand Met.	000000
Somerset County Council	B.A.T. Industries	000000
	Grand Met.	000000
	Imperial Group	000000
South Glamorgan County Council	Grand Met.	000000
	Imperial Group	000000
Staffordshire County Council	Imperial Group	000000
States of Jersey	Grand Met.	000000
Surrey County Council	B.A.T. Industries	000000
	Grand Met.	000000
	Imperial Group	000000
Tayside Regional Council	Grand Met.	000000
	Imperial Group	000000
Treasurer of the Isle of Man	B.A.T. Industries	000000
	Grand Met.	000000
Warwickshire County Council	B.A.T. Industries	000000
West Sussex County Council	Imperial Group	000000
West Midlands County Council	Molins	000000
West Yorkshire Metropolitan County Council	Imperial Group	0000000

13. EXAMPLES OF PENSION FUNDS RECORDED AS HOLDING SHARES IN THE TOBACCO INDUSTRY, AT SEPTEMBER 1984

Pension funds represent employees' earnings held in trust, and include contributions from employers and employees alike. Large investments are made, inevitably sometimes on behalf of employees who would prefer to avoid investment in tobacco. In some cases, such investments also conflict with the professional objectives of the employees concerned. The relatively few pension funds identified suggest heavy investment through nominees.

Investor	Investment in	Size of Holding
Birmingham Post and Mail Staff Pension Fund	Rothmans	000000
Co-operative Pension Funds Unit Trust Nominees	Bunzl	000000
	B.A.T. Industries	0000000
Express & Star Group Pension Scheme Ltd (Wolverhampton)	Bunzl	00000
General and Municipal Workers Pension Trustees	Grand Met.	00000
Imperial Group Pension Investments Ltd	Molins	000000
	Bunzl	000000
Imperial Group Pension Trust	Rothmans	00000
Medical Sickness Group Pension Scheme[*]	Imperial Group	00000
NCB Pension Fund Nominees	Grand Met.	00000000
	Molins	000000
	B.A.T. Industries	00000000
Penguin Pension Trustees	Rothmans	0000
Port Employers and Registered Dockworkers Pension Fund Trustees	Imperial Group	0000000

Investor	Investment in	Size of Holding
Royal National Pension Fund for Nurses[*]	Imperial Group	000000
	B.A.T. Industries	000000
	Grand Met.	000000
Royal Seamen's Pension Fund	Imperial Group	00000
States of Jersey Public Employees Pension Fund	Grand Met.	00000
University of Liverpool Pension Fund Trustees Ltd	Grand Met.	
UK Civil Service Benefit Societies Trustees Ltd	Grand Met.	00000

14. EXAMPLES OF AGENCIES/INSTITUTION IN HEALTH AND RELATED AREAS WHICH HELD SHARES IN TOBACCO COMPANIES IN 1982/3 BUT WHICH HAD SOLD SHARES BY SEPTEMBER 1984

For general comparative purposes, a record was made of share sales by organizations involved in health and related areas. No attempt was made to find out whether these organizations had made a conscious decision not to invest in tobacco—or whether shares were disposed of only for financial reasons. However, comparison with the list of health-related organizations still holding shares in tobacco (i.e. area health authorities) suggests that some organizations have decided against investment, on health-related grounds. It is possible that some organizations may not have purchased shares themselves, but may have inherited them as part of a bequest.

Investor	Investment in	Size of Holding
Barnsley Area Health Authority	Imperial Group	Nil (0000)
British Diabetic Association	B.A.T. Industries	Nil (00000)
British Institute of Radiology	Grand Met.	Nil (00)
Cancer Research Campaign	B.A.T. Industries Rothmans	Nil (0000) Nil (000)
Canterbury & Thanet Area Health Authority	B.A.T. Industries Molins	Nil (0000) Nil (0000)
Cardiff Institute for the Blind	Imperial Group	Nil (0000)
Central Manchester Health Authority Endowment Fund	B.A.T. Industries	Nil (0000)
City and East London Area Health Authority	Imperial Group	Nil
City & Hackney Health Authority	Imperial Group	Nil
General Welfare of the Blind Pension Trustees Ltd	B.A.T. Industries	Nil (00000)
Governors and Guardians of Dr Steevens Hospital, Dublin	Bunzl Imperial Group	Nil (00) Nil (0000)
Greenwich & Bexley Area Health Authority	Imperial Group	Nil (0000)
Help the Aged	Imperial Group	Nil (0000)
Incorporated Association for Promoting the General Welfare of the Blind	Grand Met. Imperial Group	Nil (0000) Nil (0000)
Institute of Orthopaedics	Imperial Group	Nil (0000)
Insitution of Ophthalmology	Imperial Group	Nil
Kent Area Health Authority	Molins	Nil (00000)
King Edward VII Hospital	B.A.T. Industries	Nil (00000)
Kirklees Area Health Authority	Imperial Group	Nil
The Mental Aftercare Association	B.A.T. Industries Imperial Group	Nil (00) Nil (000)
Middlesex Association for the Blind	Imperial Group	Nil (0000)
Norfolk Area Health Authority	Imperial Group	Nil

Investor	Investment in	Size of Holding
North England Council for the British Empire Cancer Campaign for Research	Imperial Group	Nil
Royal College of Physicians and Surgeons of Glasgow	Grand Met.	Nil (0000)
Royal College of Radiologists	Grand Met.	Nil (00)
Royal National Institute for the Blind	B.A.T. Industries	
Royal Society of Medicine	Grand Met.	Nil (00)
Somerset Area Health Authority	Imperial Group	Nil
Society for the Study of Addiction	B.A.T. Industries	Nil (00000)

15. DISCUSSION

Present levels of investment in tobacco companies cannot be reconciled with overwhelming evidence of the damaging effects of tobacco smoking on health. The extent of investment in tobacco by organizations otherwise committed to promoting good health suggests that investment decision-making is still very largely influenced by commercial factors. Major institutional investors appear as likely to invest in tobacco as in other sectors.

Having said that, divestment of shares in tobacco is not necessarily the most effective way of curbing the promotion of tobacco. In the USA, for example, selling out is considered one of the least effective things that shareholders can do—though divestment is clearly preferable to holding shares and taking no action at all.

We list here a dozen devices available for shareholder response to corporate activity considered socially harmful, in a roughly ascending order of aggressiveness:

1. Declining to invest.
2. Divestment.
3. Posing questions to management or urging management to change its policies in certain respects.

4. Withholding proxies (i.e. votes) from management or abstaining on certain socially-related resolutions proposed by other shareholders.
5. Voting in opposition to management on such resolutions.
6. Voting to unseat management in favour of opposition slates (resolutions) proposed by other stockholders.
7. Undertaking to propose the resolutions or slates referred to in items 5 and 6 on the shareholder's own initiative.
8. Soliciting proxies from other shareholders in order to carry out item 7.
9. Joining other shareholders who are bringing litigation (derivative or individual) to enjoin certain corporate conduct.
10. Bringing the litigation referred to in item 9 on the shareholders own initiative.
11. Taking any of the actions listed above pursuant to an agreement for concerted action with other shareholders.
12. Making public announcements in connection with any of the actions listed above.'

Simon, J. G., Powers, C. W. and Gunnemann, J. P. *The Ethical Investor* (New Haven, Conn.: Yale University Press, 1972).

Cultural differences between the USA and the UK, also differences in the rights and responsibilities of shareholders defined in company law, go some way to explaining the traditional lack of assertiveness of shareholders in the UK. It is still worth bearing in mind that existing and 'partly dissident' investors in tobacco, if united, represent a potentially formidable force.

Co-ordination of initiatives by shareholders should also prove worthwhile. Opportunities for achieving this could be made both through further research and by campaigning. For example, further research might be done in the following areas:

- Comprehensive searching of the registers of shareholders in tobacco companies.
- Specific enquiries into the nature and extent of undisclosed shareholdings (i.e. through nominees).
- Surveys of the investment policies of different organizations, leading to decisions not to invest, or to invest, or to divest shares in tobacco.
- Surveys of the levels of awareness and attitudes of those holding shares in tobacco—including those on whose behalf such investments are made.

- Enquiries into the availability of socially useful investments, likely to yield comparable financial returns.

Research into these and other areas are likely to create many opportunities for campaigning. Options include, for example:

- Publishing and publicizing information about the involvement of different companies in the promotion of tobacco smoking—in the UK and abroad.
- Communication with selected shareholders, inviting them to reconsider their investment position.
- Co-ordination of representations both by shareholders, and by people on whose behalf investments in tobacco are made.
- Other activities, along the lines suggested in items 1–12 above.

Any attempt to reform company behaviour through shareholder action has its limitations. On the other hand, there seems to be limitless scope for action in this area, as a means of drawing attention to the main issues.

Whatever course of action is thought most appropriate, it should be recognized, that it has been many years since the tobacco industry has raised money through the City.

The industry does not depend on investment by shareholders either to operate or expand its business.

That is not the point. The point is that an investment in tobacco can reward investors only if the industry succeeds in promoting the use of its products. To this extent, a 'good' investment means bad health.

Chapter 5

DOES TOBACCO SPORTS SPONSORSHIP ON TELEVISION ACT AS ADVERTISING TO CHILDREN?*

Frank Ledworth, PhD, Research Fellow, Department of Education, University of Manchester

A representative survey of 880 children in first, third and fifth years was carried out in five secondary schools in one education authority using an anonymous questionnaire. It was found that children were most aware of the cigarette brands which are most frequently associated with sponsored sporting events on TV. Children's TV viewing of a recent snooker championship sponsored by one cigarette manufacturer was positively correlated with the proportion of children associating that brand, and other brands used in TV sponsorship, with sport. Following a snooker championship sponsored by another cigarette manufacturer, a second survey was carried out on a new sample showing that awareness of this brand, and the proportion of children associating it with sport, had increased from the first survey. This demonstrates that the TV sports sponsorship by tobacco manufacturers acts as cigarette advertising to children and therefore circumvents the law banning cigarette advertisements on TV.

The law banning the TV advertising of cigarettes was implemented in Britain in 1965 following the failure of the tobacco companies to honour a voluntary agreement aimed at protecting children by not advertising before 9 p.m. However there has been, in recent years, a rapid growth in TV sports sponsorship by cigarette manufacturers

---

*This article first appeared in *Health Education Journal*, **43**(4), 1984, and is reproduced here with permission.

which might have an influence on children. There is evidence from Australia[1] that children's cigarette brand preferences are more heavily concentrated than adults' preferences on the brand which is most frequently promoted by sponsorship on TV.

There is a need for details of the effects of sports sponsorship, bearing in mind the views quoted by the advertising industry's own press that: 'the Embassy (snooker championship on TV) . . . must rank as the media buy of the century (which) coupled with the high cost of airtime and the growing restrictions on advertising of tobacco . . . is forcing more and more companies to consider sponsorship as a serious part of their marketing plans.[2] Any evidence that such tobacco sports sponsorship acts as advertising would indicate that it circumvents the above mentioned law. For such a case to be made it is not necessary (nor was this intended here) to demonstrate any link between sponsorship and children's smoking behaviour. As indicated below this is a wider issue which requires further study. The present investigation was intended to be the first step in such a process.

The aim of the present study was to investigate in children whether exposure to two tobacco-sponsored sports events on BBC TV appeared to act as advertising. This was defined as activities which increase the level of awareness of certain brands and the association in children's minds of these brands with an attractive activity, in this case sport.

There were problems in the design of the study since it is impossible to establish a baseline of knowledge in children not exposed to tobacco sponsorship since such promotion is all-pervasive. Therefore two surveys of cigarette brand awareness in children were carried out: the first after the televising of a snooker championship sponsored by Benson and Hedges (B&H), and the second after the televising of a snooker championship sponsored by Embassy. Different children were used in the surveys to avoid the contaminating effect of sensitizing children to the information sought.

THE FIRST SURVEY

Method

A two-stage sampling method was used. The sampling frame consisted of all state-funded secondary schools in one education authority in the Greater Manchester area. A random sample of five schools was drawn and, at the second stage, a random sample was drawn of 11 classes from the complete list of classes for the first, third and fifth years separately. The survey was carried out from 13–24 February 1984, that is between two and three weeks after the end of the Benson & Hedges Masters Snooker Championship which received 28 hours of coverage on BBC TV. All the children in the sample were tested as intact classes by their form teacher using an anonymous questionnaire sealed into one envelope for the whole class on completion. No attempt was made to follow up the 46 (5 per cent) absentees. The children were asked to list the cigarette brands they knew, their smoking habits, intentions and attitudes, and the extent of their viewing of the recent snooker championship. Differences in the number of cigarette brands recalled were analysed by analysis of variance and differences in proportions recalling particular brands by chi square test.

Results

There were 880 children tested with year and sex break down as shown in Table 1. There was an over-representation of boys but the proportions admitting smoking (at least occasionally) were not signi-ficantly different $\chi^2 = 6.52$, 3df) from national estimates: the numbers were 9 (three per cent), 68 (23 per cent) and 101 (36 per cent) at first, third and fifth year as compared with two per cent, 15 per cent and 36 per

TABLE 1   The sample: by school year and sex

Year	1st year 11–12 years	3rd year 13–14 years	5th year 15–16 years	Total
n	301	295	281	880
(%)	(34)	(34)	(32)	
Year not recorded = 3				
Sex	Boys	Girls		
n	494	381		880
(%)	(56)	(44)		
Sex not recorded = 5				

cent found in a nationally representative survey with follow-up of absentees.[3]

Only 13 (1.5 per cent) of the children failed to list any cigarette brand. The mean number of brands recalled was 5.5 and was higher in older children ($p<0.001$), in regular smokers ($p<0.001$) and in those

TABLE 2   References to individual cigarette brands

	BH	JPS	EM	P6	PD	SC	MAR	PS	WB	Base
Brand listed first	497 (57)	98 (11)	82 (9)	19 (2)	28 (3)	45 (5)	30 (3)	5 (1)	4 (—)	880 (%)
Brand listed at all	780 (89)	632 (72)	535 (61)	187 (21)	238 (27)	429 (49)	226 (26)	136 (16)	63 (7)	880 (%)
Preferred brand among smokers	138 (76)	10 (6)	16 (9)	3 (2)	— (—)	8 (4)	5 (3)	1 (—)	— (—)	181 (%)
Brands associated with sport	337 (38)	347 (39)	240 (27)	2 (—)	2 (—)	7 (—)	121 (14)	3 (—)	0 (—)	880 (%)
Brand named as sponsor of snooker	275 (31)	20 (2)	221 (25)	0 (—)	0 (—)	2 (—)	0 (—)	0 (—)	0 (—)	880 (%)
Hours of TV sponsored sport source (1983)[a]	73	43	132	—	—	11.0	8.0	2.0	—	
Market % brand share (1982)[b]	16	13	21.8	4.3	2.0	7.0	2.25	3.0	1.5	
Advertising expenditure (1983) (£M)[c]	7.3	5.2	5.2	76	nk	5.4	25	1.0	nk	

Key   BH = Benson & Hedges   JPS = John Player Special
       EM = Embassy   P6 = Players No 6
       PD = Park Drive   SC = Silk Cut
       MAR = Marlboro   PS = Peter Stuyvesant
       WB = Woodbine

Sources
[a] Sports Sponsorship Computer Analyses Ltd
[b] Tobacco September 1983
[c] MEAL Quarterly Digest, 4th Quarter, 1983

who intended to smoke in the future ($p < 0.005$), whether they were current smokers or not.

Table 2 shows that one brand, B&H, was predominant amongst the first brand listed. Of the brands listed at all, the three best known were B&H, John Player Special (JPS) and Embassy. To the question: 'If you smoke, write down the brand or brands you prefer to smoke', 181 pupils replied and the choice of the great majority of these was B&H. The question was asked: 'Are there any sports you connect with particular brands of cigarette? If so write down the name of the cigarette brand and next to it the sport or sports you link it with'. There were only four cigarette brands frequently associated with sport, with two, B&H and JPS, being most prominent.

Conversely there were only four sports linked with any substantial frequency with cigarette brands: snooker (435 children, 49 per cent), motor racing (342, 39 per cent), cricket (98, 11 per cent) and darts (52, 6 per cent). The table shows that two brands were thought to have sponsored the recent snooker: B&H, the actual sponsors and Embassy, which has more hours of sponsored snooker, taking the year as a whole. For comparison the last three rows show respectively the hours of sports sponsorship exposure, the share of adult sales of the tobacco brands listed and the total advertising revenue.

Children were asked 'On how many days did you watch the Masters Championship snooker on TV recently'. Only 232 children (26 per cent) did not watch at all, 314 (36 per cent) watched one day, 198 (23 per cent) watched two to seven days and (125 (14 per cent) watched 8 days or more. As Table 3 shows, children who watched more snooker

TABLE 3   Number and percentage of references to cigarette brands linked with sport and amount of snooker watched

Cigarette brand linked with sport	Amount of snooker watched				χ^2 (3df)
	Not at all	1–2 days	3–7 days	8 days or more	
B&H	52(22)	116(37)	94(48)	74(59)	54.9*
JPS	56(24)	126(40)	103(52)	60(48)	39.6*
Embassy	20 (9)	77(25)	77(39)	65(52)	93.4*
Marlboro	26(11)	45(14)	30(15)	19(15)	1.9
Base:	232	314	198	125	

Snooker watching not recorded: 11
*$p < 0.001$

were more likely to associate various cigarette brands with sport, particularly B&H, JPS and Embassy, the three brands with the greatest exposure in terms of TV sport sponsorship.

Discussion

The data showed that the majority of the children had seen the sponsored snooker and that the cigarette brands which were best known to the children and most associated by them with sports were those which are most heavily promoted by TV sports sponsorship. There was thus some evidence to support the suggestion that such sponsorship acts as advertising in informing about tobacco brands and linking these with sport. The supplementary evidence that children who watched more snooker on TV were more likely to link B&H and several other brands with sport suggests that there may be a general 'sports-linkage' effect of watching tobacco-sponsored sport on TV, in addition to the specific effects of any one event.

However, the evidence was only correlational—children who watch a great deal of sport on TV may not be typical—and thus the evidence should only be used with caution to suggest a causal link between TV sponsored sports viewing and an advertising effect. In addition there was the possible confounding effect that the brands best known to the children were also those most widely sold and advertised. However, the Embassy brand name was relatively less known and less associated with sport than would be expected on the basis of brand market share and exposure in TV sports sponsorship.

It was hypothesized that Embassy was less familiar and less associated with sport since it had not had recent exposure through sports sponsorship on TV. A second survey was therefore carried out in the week following the end of the Embassy World Snooker Championship, which had over 100 hours of TV coverage from 21 April to May 7 1984. The aim of this second survey was to examine the extent of any differences from the first survey in awareness of the Embassy brand and in its association with sport.

THE SECOND SURVEY

Of the five schools in the original survey only three were available for re-testing due to problems of industrial action. In addition the fifth year pupils were no longer in school on a regular basis. Therefore the same number of classes were selected at random from each of the three schools in each of the first and third years as had been tested in the first survey, with the restriction that no class was tested a second time. The questionnaire contained the same questions as in the first survey, with the addition of three extra questions, which were placed last so that most of the questionnaire was the same as in the first survey. Conditions of testing were the same as in the first survey, with the whole class of children completing the anonymous questionnaire in one session, supervised by the class teacher, the answers being sealed into an envelope on completion.

Results

There were no significant differences between the two surveys as to break down by age group, school or smoking habits, but there was an increased proportion of girls in the second survey as Table 4 shows. There were more absentees in the second survey—71 children (21 per cent), with the proportion varying from 2/30 to 10/26 in different classes. In the second survey 188 children (69 per cent) reported having watched the snooker, with 57 (21 per cent) reporting viewing on 8 days or more. Some 119 children (44 per cent) correctly identified Embassy as the sponsoring brand, with a further 31 (11 per cent) naming B&H.

Table 5 shows that the second survey found no increase in the proportion of children recalling B&H but there was an increase in the recall of Embassy. Amongst girls there was a statistically significantly greater increase ($p<0.001$) in the proportion recalling Embassy—16.9 percentage points in girls as compared with 7.9 percentage points in boys. There was also an increase in the proportion listing Marlboro and, to a lesser extent, JPS.

The proportion of children linking Embassy with sport more than doubled—as Table 6 shows. The change in boys was 28.1 percentage points compared with 21.9 percentage points in girls. The results on brand awareness and linkage of particular brands with sports were not statistically significantly different for classes above and below the median level of absenteeism, suggesting that this later factor had not influenced the observed differences in brand awareness and association with sport between the first and second surveys. It should be noted that with both sexes combined there was a greatly increased association of both JPS and Marlboro with sports.

TABLE 4   Sample profiles from the first and second surveys by school year, sex and smoking status

	School Year		School No.			Sex		Smoking status		
	1	3	1	2	4	M	F	never	experimented	regular
First survey n (%)	163 (50.2)	162 (49.8)	88 (27.1)	56 (17.2)	181 (55.7)	144 (44.4)	180 (55.6)	150 (47.2)	118 (37.1)	50 (15.7)
Second survey n (%)	145 (53.3)	127 (46.7)	73 (26.8)	48 (17.6)	151 (55.5)	88 (33.9)	171 (66.0)	132 (49.1)	111 (41.3)	26 (9.7)
χ^2	<1		<1			6.58 (1df)		4.88 (2df)		
p						<0.02		NS		

Base
First survey 325
Second survey 272

Not recorded
First survey: Smoking 7, Sex 1
Second survey: Smoking 3, Sex 13

TABLE 5   Frequency (percentage) of brands mentioned in the first and second surveys

	Brand							
	BH	JPS	EM	P6	PD	SC	MAR	PS
First survey	283 (87.1)	209 (64.3)	179 (55.1)	77 (23.7)	95 (29.2)	144 (44.3)	47 (14.5)	38 (11.7)
Second survey	243 (89.3)	193 (70.9)	186 (68.4)	61 (22.4)	91 (33.5)	133 (48.9)	76 (27.9)	29 (10.7)
Change (% points)	+2.2	+6.6	+13.3	−1.5	+4.3	+4.6	+13.4	−1.0
χ^2(1df)	<1	2.98	11.0	<1	1.23	1.25	16.5	<1
p	NS	NS	<0.001	<1	NS	NS	<0.001	<1

Base: First Survey 325   Second Survey 272

TABLE 6 Frequency (percentage) of cigarette brands associated with sports: comparison of first and second surveys

	BH	JPS	EM	P6	PD	SC	MAR	PS
First survey	88 (27.1)	86 (26.5)	58 (17.8)	0 (—)	0 (—)	1 (0.3)	18 (5.5)	0
Second survey	92 (33.8)	123 (45.2)	111 (40.8)	3 (1.1)	0 (—)	5 (1.8)	45 (16.5)	0
Change	+6.7	+18.7	+23.0	+1.1	—	+1.5	+11.0	—
χ^2	3.20	22.9	38.47	<1	—	<1	19.0	—
p	NS	<0.001	<0.001	<0.001	—		<0.001	—

Base: First Survey 325   Second Survey 272

DISCUSSION

There seems to be no reasonable doubt that the increase for the Embassy brand in knowledge and association with sport between the two surveys could be attributed, at least in part, to exposure to sponsored snooker on TV immediately prior to the second survey. The two samples were drawn from the same schools and age groups and there were no significant changes in awareness of the B&H brand which, in a sense, acted as the control brand.

In so far as there were any differences, there were somewhat fewer smokers in the second survey. Since smokers tend to know more brands it would have been expected that awareness of Embassy and other brands would have been lower in the second survey. Differences in the proportions by sex and the higher rate of absenteeism in the second survey would not appear to have determined the results since the differences in brand awareness were shown (though not to the same degree) in boys and girls and the level of absenteeism had no effect on brand awareness and linkage with sport.

The increased knowledge of Marlboro and its linkage, together with JPS, with sport, are noteworthy and indicate the problems of carrying out before and after studies outside the laboratory when all other factors cannot necessarily be held constant. In the interval between the two surveys, there were two Grand Prix motor racing events shown on BBC TV and several Grandstand TV programmes featured motor racing. The Marlboro and JPS racing cars figured prominently in these events and their pictures were widely used to publicize the events, even in *Radio Times*, which does not accept paid cigarette advertising. The increase in awareness of the sponsored brands suggests that even fairly brief exposure to tobacco-sponsored sports on TV, if linked to well-publicised images, may produce a considerable increase in levels of brand awareness and association with sport.

Given the definition of advertising suggested above—activities which familiarize the audience with the name of a brand and associate it with positive images or ideas—it must be concluded that the sponsorship on TV by the manufacturers of Embassy acted as advertising to children. Thus the sponsorship appeared to circumvent both the law banning cigarette advertising on TV, and the BBC Licence and Agreement which (in Clause 12) states that: the BBC 'shall not send or emit . . . any sponsored programme' and (in Clause 13) forbids 'the transmission of television images of very brief duration which "might convey a message to . . . the minds of an audience without them being aware, or fully aware, of what has been done" '.[4]

There is a need for further investigation to determine whether tobacco sports sponsorship not only acts as advertising as defined earlier, but also persuades children to smoke. The studies (which are equivocal) as to whether tobacco promotion does encourage people to smoke are not directly relevant to the question of the effects on children. Such studies are based on econometric analyses[5,6] and deal with aggregate demand (of which children's smoking accounts for no more than 1 or 2 billion[7] of the total of 102 billion per year[8]). A large change in the prevalence of smoking in children would have a negligible impact on aggregate demand but might have a major influence on future smoking prevalence since most regular smokers adopt the habit before the age of 18.[9] Moreover it should be noted that econometric studies only examine advertising expenditure and ignore sponsorship which is small in terms of money but, the present evidence suggests, may be disproportionately effective in its impact on children.

We need more detailed longitudinal studies of the impact of various types of tobacco promotion on the behaviour of representative samples of children, although it should be born in mind that longitudinal studies are unlikely to breach anonymity and thus lead to problems in the under-reporting of smoking. Recently announced government-commissioned research using small group discussions, which it is thought, 'could even disclose that sports sponsorship . . . may have no effect in persuading young people to smoke',[10] have little of substance to offer. Few people would admit that advertising affects their behaviour, yet there is no doubt of the aggregate effect of advertising on sales.

For the present it is contended that the case rests that sports sponsorship on BBC TV has been shown to act as cigarette advertising to children. There would thus appear to be good grounds for calling for the cessation of tobacco sports sponsorship on TV so as to prevent further circumvention of the law banning the TV advertising of cigarettes.

ACKNOWLEDGEMENTS

I wish to thank David Whicker and Peter Taylor of BBC *Panorama* who gave encouragement and financial support for the first survey, the Director of Education, head teachers and children who made it possible to carry out the surveys, Mrs M. Ali and Ms D. McCool who helped with the data preparation and analysis and The Health Education Council who funded my Research Fellowship.

REFERENCES

1. Chapman, S. and Fitzgerald, B. *American Journal of Public Health*, 1981, **73**, 492.
2. Koski, J. *Campaign*, 1981, 28 August.
3. Dobbs, J. and Marsh, A. *Smoking Among Secondary School Children*, London: HMSO, 1983.
4. *BBC Annual Report and Handbook 1984*, BBC, 1984; 173–174.
5. McGuinness, T. and Cowling, K. *European Economic Review*, July 1975.
6. Metra Consulting Group Ltd. *The relationship between total cigarette advertising and total cigarette consumption in the UK*, 1979.
7. Dobbs, J. and Marsh, A. See Ref. 3, p. 19.
8. *Tobacco*, September, 1983.
9. Marsh, A. and Matheson, J. *Smoking Attitudes and Behaviour*, London: HMSO, 1983.
10. Russell, W. *British Medical Journal*, 1984; **289**, 60.

INDEX